FAITH
IN HOSPICES

FAITH IN HOSPICES

Spiritual Care and the End of Life

_____

Derek Murray

Published in Great Britain in 2002 by
Society for Promoting Christian Knowledge
Holy Trinity Church
Marylebone Road
London NW1 4DU

The author and publisher acknowledge with thanks
permission to reproduce material from
Bruce Rumbold: *Helplessness and Hope*: SCM Press, 1986.

Every effort has been made to trace and acknowledge the copyright
holder of 'Fisher Jamie' by John Buchan, in W. H. Hamilton (ed.),
Holyrood: A Garland of Modern Scots Poems, Dent. If notified,
the publisher will ensure that a full acknowledgement is made
in a subsequent edition of this book.

British Library Cataloguing-in-Publication Data
A catalogue record for this book is available
from the British Library

ISBN 0-281-05228-X

Typeset by Pioneer Associates, Perthshire
Printed in Great Britain by
The Cromwell Press, Trowbridge, Wiltshire

To Giles,
teacher and friend

Contents

Preface

I came into the hospice world by what at the time seemed an accident. I was profoundly ignorant of what might be in store. Twenty-three years later I have reached retirement. This book is a reflection on these years and on the very remarkable movement that has, from the beginning, been inspired by clear Christian principles and in the case of many who lead it, by clear Christian commitment.

The strains that affect all the churches have not left the hospice movement untouched or unchanged. In a secular society the need for sensitive care of the dying remains great and, indeed, may be said to have increased in intensity, as families can seem less stable and supportive. I write as a chaplain and therefore with evident bias. I hope that this book will help clergy and others to think creatively about the care of the dying and that it will contribute to this essential ministry of Christ's Church.

Derek B. Murray
Edinburgh, November 2001

Acknowledgements

My debts are many, as ministry in the hospice has so many aspects. I would like to thank my family and the Baptist churches at Dublin Street (now Canonmills) and Morningside, Edinburgh, for their support and encouragement. Dr David Lyall and Professor Alastair Campbell suggested that I might apply for the post of Chaplain at St Columba's Hospice and have been constant sources of inspiration and friendship ever since. The Revd Stuart Coates, the Revd Tom Gordon and many other hospice chaplains have accompanied me and taught me. Dr Derek Doyle, Medical Director of St Columba's Hospice 1977–95 guided and cajoled me into unfamiliar fields of study and supported my ministry, as did so many members of staff, volunteers, patients and families over the years. Thank you.

CHAPTER ONE

The Hospice Movement

In late 1993 a retired teacher with the unusual Christian name of Giles realized that she had not been invited for her three-yearly appointment at the Breast Screening Clinic. She called in and was told that it was assumed that she was male because of her name, and that men did not always appreciate being contacted by that clinic. So she was examined amidst some laughter, only to be told a few days later to return, as there was a lump. Then followed fear, anger, anxiety, and renewed hope after a lumpectomy and radiotherapy. She and her husband were able to go to Cyprus and Egypt to celebrate their 35th wedding anniversary. A referral was made to the hospice Home Care service, as it was then known, so that any problems could be addressed.

In the autumn of 1994 Giles began to feel tired and developed a variety of pains. After tests 'something was found in the blood' and from then on the decline in health was rapid. At the end of January 1995 the hospice Home Care sister called, and sent for the Medical Director. Within a few hours Giles was admitted to the hospice, clutching her Bible and Tolkien's *The Lord of the Rings*, which she was rereading. Suddenly she became confused from time to time, to the distress of her husband and two adult daughters, although she was able to set her funeral arrangements in order, and to talk lucidly to the friend and actor who had agreed to give her eulogy. She became unconscious and, one week after entering the hospice, she died during the night.

If I had wanted to invent a paradigm for hospice care, this might be it. Excellent service from experienced practitioners, good co-ordination with the general practice, a short admission, with some time for the family to visit and say farewell, enough clarity of mind to plan the funeral, right down to the music and the organists who were to play in church and crematorium. But it is not quite so straightforward. Giles was my wife and I had already been a hospice chaplain for 17 years. We both knew too much and too little. I have made things sound calm and inevitable but they were not. Giles had been born with mild cerebral palsy which had not deterred her from motherhood and a career in teaching. She had triumphed bravely over a real disability, and she had a lively and experimental faith. She believed in intercessory prayer, and it worked. But when the first diagnosis was made she was angry – with the clinic, with God, with the Devil, and with me for not understanding. She screamed and I sent for a good friend as I didn't know how to deal with this fury. Gradually she worked through her anger, and in a brief autobiography which I was able to print off the computer after her death, she said 'I asked "why me?" and then very gradually I was able to say "why not me?"' The funeral was a wonderful mixture of sadness and triumph. She had indeed 'fought the good fight'.

As for me, I went in to work at the hospice the day she was admitted, ready to visit the patients. I was sent home, after giving the names of six local clergy who would cover one day each for me. I tried to become a visitor. I had the support of our two daughters and of many family members and friends. I thought I coped. The Medical Director was anxious about me. I found an outlet in writing and in talking about Giles and about what had happened, and in three weeks I was so bored at home that I went back to work, and wept in private. I do not recommend such an experience to other hospice chaplains, but I have seen our institution from many angles, and I hope that my own involvement in loss and grief, and my days as a visitor, have made me open to the fears and needs of others.

Everyone seems to know about hospices, but there is more to tell and discuss. There may be a need for a view of the hospice movement and the questions it raises from the chaplain's perspective. This book will try to address one of the most recent developments in medical care, which has arisen first in the United Kingdom and then spread to many other parts of the world. The hospice appears in novels and plays, in soap operas and Acts of Parliament. Although it has relatively few beds and gives at best a patchy coverage, even in its home in Great Britain, yet many people have been affected by it. Some have blessed it and some have deplored its existence, but it is hard to ignore. The modern hospice movement dates only from the 1960s, although it did not appear *ex nihilo*, and it is perhaps too soon to give a definitive appreciation of its work. It began in the Christian Churches, and has spread far beyond. It is, then, important to assess the place of faith and of chaplaincy in the hospice movement, and that I will try to do in the next few chapters.

There are so many books and articles about death and dying that it may seem unnecessary and perhaps presumptuous to produce yet another. At least since the early 1970s death and dying have been favourite subjects for doctors, nurses, sociologists, historians and theologians to investigate, although theologians and pastors have, of course, been interested in the subject for much longer. The dying process seems to be a preoccupation of late modernity. As in the developed countries, people have expected to live longer and more healthily, so attention has been turned to the inevitable but mysterious subject of the end of life.

Death and dying, while occasions of sadness and regret, were nevertheless accepted as inevitable, and were a shared communal experience in most communities until the very recent modern period. The great civilizations of the Ancient Near East produced elaborate tombs for rulers and for their immediate servants and families, but the death of the ordinary peasant seems to have passed almost unnoticed. It was part of the natural order, and the vividly portrayed after-life journey was for the great and good. Even in the Old Testament, death stories are mostly about kings and their families, although there are also accounts of the death and revival of widows' sons. Death is simply accepted as a natural event, being 'gathered to one's fathers', and life went on in the surviving generations. Such ideas of immortality as there are

in the Old Testament very largely concern living on through
one's descendants. Ideas of personal immortality and bodily
resurrection are generally considered to have entered Hebrew
religion after the Exile to Babylon in the sixth century BCE,
and to have become widespread only in the last two centuries
before Christ. In Christianity life after death plays a central
role. A faith based on a dying and rising Lord can scarcely
ignore the afterlife, and most expressions of Christian theology
treat the subject, sometimes in very different ways. Some
interpretations of Judaism look forward to life after death, but
generally immortality is not of so much concern to Jews as it
is to Christians and indeed to Muslims.

The privatization of death in Western civilization, of which
Ariès writes in *The Hour of Our Death*, is quite recent, and we
can still be shocked at the apparent nonchalance with which
people in the eighteenth and nineteenth centuries accepted
the death of their loved ones. In the 1770s Mrs Thrale, the
friend of Dr Johnson, remarked when a daughter died within
ten hours of birth, 'one cannot grieve after her much, and I
have just now other things to think on'. Lawrence Stone goes
on to comment that 'the modern association of death with the
aged bears no relation to reality at any earlier period, when
relatively few died at a ripe old age'.[1]

In a roll book of a small Baptist church in Glasgow for the
early years of the nineteenth century, there are two references
to death in childbed on one page, and surprise is only
expressed at the death of Samuel Ferguson in September
1834. 'Died very suddenly of cholera. Attended his wife's
funeral on Saturday in perfect health – at work on Monday
and died on Tuesday.'[2] Life and the human hold on it were
very much more tenuous in the recent past than we like to
remember. In an article in the *British Medical Journal* for 1933
David Rorie, a general practitioner and folklorist in rural
Scotland, remarks that 'the value set on human life has varied
in the past and may vary further in the future, but inherent
in mankind is the quite understandable belief that this value
lessens with age'. Talking of forty years before his time he
asserts that 'various things indicate that the lives of the senile,
the decrepit, the sick who were a danger to others, and the

deformed child were held to be of small account'. The article is entitled 'Hastening the Death of the Aged, Infirm and Sick'.[3] It is unlikely that such an article would find a respected journal to publish it today, yet Rorie bases his writing on experience and folk-wisdom. It may be that only recently has an absolute value been set on human life, thus creating a climate for the development of the hospice movement.

At the same time as death was an ever-present threat, talk about it was commonplace, and although it was feared, it was also named. Gorer, in 1955,[4] proclaimed that death was the great taboo, and it has become almost trite to say that while sex was the subject that Victorians avoided, for modern people death had become the great secret. What had happened? Later we will discuss the medicalization of death and the changes in social expectations and in family life. Here it can be said that generalizations are very dangerous and likely to need many modifications. There have always been speculations and beliefs about death, and the changes noted in recent history may not be as significant as they appear. What we can say for certain is that since 1955 when Gorer wrote, the volume of books and articles concerning death and dying has been increasing at an alarming rate, and that since around the same time the concept of hospice care has evolved from a minority interest into an accepted medical and social phenomenon in the English-speaking world and far beyond. How far the hospice movement has influenced the attitudes of society, and how far it has been shaped by its environment, are matters that may become clearer as we go on.

WHAT THEN IS A HOSPICE?

So familiar is the word hospice today that I seldom have to explain what such an institution is. That does not mean that many who have never yet directly encountered a hospice have a clear idea of what it looks and feels like, and there are still many myths around and patients still arrive saying they have never heard of the place. But documentaries on television, books, references in soap operas and novels and plentiful newspaper coverage have made the word, if not the concept, extremely well known. Local hospices are often generously supported charities in their communities. One has only to compare the experience of collecting in a busy street for the hospice with days spent feeling invisible or resented when shaking a can for an overseas aid charity to realize the popularity and acceptability of this relatively recent form of care. People cross the road to push a cheque into the tin, and very few pass indifferently!

Where does this seemingly new idea come from? When St Columba's Hospice opened in Edinburgh in 1977 there was another hospice round the corner, a retirement home belonging to the Order of St John of Jerusalem, which has since moved to a new location. This led to confusion, but the word was being used for a caring institution. After the First World War Dr Elsie Inglis, famous for her medical exploits during the war and for her work for mothers and babies in the city, opened a hospice in the High Street of Edinburgh, to care for single mothers. The association with dying people, found for example in the tenth edition of the *Merriam Webster Collegiate Dictionary*, is relatively recent. It reads: '1. A lodging for travellers, young persons, or the underprivileged, esp. when maintained by a religious order. 2. a facility or program designed to provide a caring environment for supplying the physical and emotional needs of the terminally ill.' The *Oxford English Dictionary* of 1933 gives two definitions, one as 'a house of rest and entertainment for pilgrims, travellers or strangers, also generally a home for the destitute or the sick,' quoting *The Times* for 18 December 1894: 'the hospice provides 20 beds, soup, bread and coals to families, and penny dinners to sandwich-men.' The other, quoting Hastings Rashdall's *Universities of Europe*, is 'a Hostel for students'. The Latin form 'hospitium' is sometimes found for either institution. So the word 'hospice' has meant an inn by the roadside, a place of care for mothers and babies, for the destitute and sick, for the elderly and for the dying.

The meaning adopted in this book is therefore relatively recent. It is customary to speak of the modern hospice movement, and to date it from the 1960s when St Christopher's Hospice in Sydenham, south London, was founded and became a paradigm for other such places. But no movement can appear without a history. The popular and rather romantic story is that there is a direct link at least as a concept with pilgrim inns in the Middle Ages, which catered for those who were travelling to Canterbury or Santiago de Compostela. The modern hospice was thus seen as the last staging post of our earthly journey, an inn by the wayside where weary travellers could find rest, refreshment and Christian worship and prayer. While this is easy to dismiss as an invented and sentimental link, it at least has its value in defining ideals of hospitality, welcome, and care that are not in any way related to profit.

The actual origins are both more simple and more complex. In the Middle Ages Christians carried on a much more ancient tradition of caring for the sick and weary traveller. The medieval hospices – whether the great fortress hospital of Rhodes, the elegant hospice of Beaune, or the myriad of small hospices associated with monasteries all over Europe – were dedicated to the care of the sick and the dying, and the Christian burial of the dead. Whether the traveller was a knight on the journey to Jerusalem, or a poor beggar on the journey of life, the ancient hospice was a way station, a resting-place, a place of care and concern for both the body and the spirit.

A Lutheran order of deaconesses was founded at Kaiserswerth, in Germany, in 1836, which had as its aim the care of the sick and the dying, and in 1842 Mme Jeanne Garnier, a Roman Catholic, founded a number of 'Calvaires', or hospices for the dying, in France. Calvary Hospital, New York, owed much to this concept. In 1879 the Sisters of Charity opened a hospice for the dying near Dublin, and went on to open St Joseph's in Hackney, London, in 1905. In 1893 St Luke's House for the Dying Poor was opened under Methodist auspices, and this became one of the places where Cicely Saunders found inspiration. Also in Clapham in London there was the Hostel of God, founded in 1891 and now renamed Trinity Hospice. It was staffed for many years by the Sisters of St Margaret's, East Grinstead. These institutions could be described as bridges between the medieval hospices and the modern movement. They were certainly inspired by Christian faith and stood in the great tradition of caring for the needy in the name of Jesus.

But they had little effect either on the general healthcare system or on public opinion. In surviving records we can read of the desire to provide a good death, although sometimes only for those who deserved it. St Luke's with its evangelical Methodist ethos was quite definitely for the 'deserving poor', who were presented with an opportunity for conversion to Christ before they died. In St Joseph's the stated aim was to provide a holy and happy death, in communion with the Catholic Church and surrounded by the symbols and rituals of the faith. The Hostel of God hoped to offer a similar possibility, in the Anglo-Catholic tradition. Although many patients had cancer, tuberculosis was the most frequent reason for the need of care, and the commonest cause of death in the nineteenth and early twentieth centuries.[5]

When Cicely Saunders set out to find a new way to care for the dying she was building on strong foundations. In 1957 she wrote her first paper, 'Dying of Cancer', which was published in the *St Thomas's Hospital Gazette*. It was based on her work in St Luke's Hospital in Bayswater, and on four case studies of cancer patients. In it she explored the value of special homes for terminally ill patients, refuting the notion that these are 'dismal and depressing places' and arguing for the advantage that 'those working in them are specialists, and from experience know how to deal with pain, fungating and eroding growths, mental distress, fear and resentment'. The question of telling the patient and relatives about the diagnosis and prognosis is discussed; the value of spiritual care is explored; details of nursing care are set out; and particular attention is given to the issue of pain management.[6]

This paper was sent to various organizations working with the dying and it elicited varied reactions. One general practitioner who visited a Marie Curie home objected to the idea of telling patients their diagnosis. He claimed that the very reverse practice was most effective but nevertheless wished her well in this 'unfortunate branch of practice'. Such reactions still occur, and references to a 'depressing place to work' are still fairly commonplace.

However most reactions were more positive and Dr Saunders, as she was then, set about gaining support and funding for the projected home, which she envisaged by 1959 as having 60 beds for terminally ill patients, with facilities for chronically sick and elderly persons, including former staff and their relatives. This foundation would be financially independent to allow freedom of action, but would expect some contractual arrangements with the National Health Service. It was seen as a form of religious community, and would be called St Christopher's Hospice. As the years went on, powerful supporters were recruited, and many charitable bodies were approached, often successfully. Underlying all the preparations was Dr Saunders' sense of God's calling. Coming as she did from an Anglican Evangelical background she was familiar with the concept of a personal task from God being set for each believer, who would be given the strength to attain it. She firmly believed in prayer, and expected answers. St Joseph's Hospice in Hackney was at the time largely staffed by the Irish Sisters of Charity, and although Dr Saunders was wary of certain elements in Roman Catholicism, she sought to set the Hospice in the same Christian tradition but firmly in the Church of England mould. Soon her personal sense of calling was extended to the institution, which she saw as something 'meant'. But the idea of religious community, despite her links with the communities at Taizé and Grandchamps, began to fade, especially as several large donors refused to support a 'unidenominational' project. The spiritual aspects of care continued to dominate her thinking: 'I long to bring patients to know the Lord and to do something about helping many to hear of Him before they die, but I also long to raise the standards of terminal care throughout the country from a medical point of view at least, even when I can do nothing about the spiritual part of the work.'[7] This quotation from a letter to the Revd Bruce Reed sums up the dilemma of the founders of the hospice movement. Which is more important, medical competence or spiritual care? That is rather a bald way of expressing it, but undoubtedly there can be tension between competence and enthusiasm in treating the dying, especially for believing staff, and the chaplain may naturally be caught up in this.

Even before St Christopher's was opened contacts had been

made throughout the United Kingdom and with professionals
who shared its aims in the United States. After 1967 the concept of the hospice spread remarkably quickly. At first there
could be, as the history of St Barnabas' Hospice in Worthing
illustrates, local opposition. In this case it came from the local
Nursing Home Association which felt its position and skills
threatened. There was also the question of finance. The Worthing Hospice, for a brief period, attempted to charge according
to patients' means, but soon abandoned this practice, and
generally speaking, in the UK, hospices have not charged
patients.[8] In the 70s and 80s hospices opened in many towns
and cities in the UK and Ireland. Dr Saunders, soon to become
Dame Cicely, was generous with her time and enthusiasm,
and other charismatic doctors and nurses spread the word. In
some respects hospices became a new missionary movement
('on the last frontier!' as a hospital chaplain remarked to me
at the beginning of St Columba's). Very soon specialist Home
Care sisters were appointed for domiciliary care, and the
Macmillan Cancer Relief Fund paid for them in their first few
years in each area. They became known as Macmillan Sisters,
or Macmillan Nurses, and even when the financing of the
service became the responsibility of the local hospice, the
designation remained. Such sisters, highly qualified and
motivated, were appointed also in areas where there was no
hospice, and were often attached to local health centres. More
recently specialist palliative care teams, comprising a doctor,
nurses, and social workers, have been set up in general hospitals, to apply the principles of care exemplified in the hospice
movement.

In Canada, Australia and New Zealand, and several other
countries, development has been similar to the UK. In the
United States, while there are a few free-standing hospices,
hospice care is mostly delivered by nurses and volunteers in
the homes of cancer patients, and this pattern is replicated in
Germany and elsewhere. In Saudi Arabia there is a Home
Care Service, and in China hospices, seen mainly as being for
the elderly, are being set up and are increasing in number.
There are programmes assisted by Western expertise and aid
in Africa and India, and links have been made with similar
work in Eastern Europe.

At the end of the twentieth century hospice and palliative care, in a form originating in the UK, had taken root in different forms in almost every part of the world. Rightly, local conditions and the availability of funding have influenced the way in which the services have developed. Germans may, so a colleague now working in a hospice in Germany informs me, remain suspicious of special places in which people die, yet in Poland, near Auschwitz-Birkenau, a large free-standing hospice has recently been opened in Krakow. There has been a danger that too many hospices with too small a financial base might be set up, and some institutions have never been able to use all their beds for lack of funds, but the more recent trend to NHS- funded palliative care teams, hospice wards in general hospitals and to Hospice-at-Home, may be a sign that the great period of building is almost over.

In Britain several free-standing units in the grounds of hospitals have come into the hospice orbit, and the Marie Curie Centres, which in earlier years were designed for longer stay patients than were general in hospices, and which sometimes had no resident doctor, have now become very similar to St Christopher-inspired hospices. In Edinburgh the catchment area for St Columba's Hospice has gradually contracted over the years. In Fife, hospice wards have opened in Dunfermline and Kirkcaldy, and Fairmile Marie Curie Centre has come to serve South Edinburgh and part of the Lothians, leaving St Columba's with North Edinburgh and the other parts of the surrounding counties. This has in no way lessened the demand for beds, but it has certainly made family visiting easier! Similar patterns can be observed in other parts of the country.

Many hospices and some general hospitals have day care units, where patients who are being looked after at home can spend one or two days per week, sharing with in-patients occupational and diversional therapy, entertainment, company and the security of knowing that the doctor and the nurse are not too far away. In due course many day care patients will enter the nursing wing, and they at least have the advantage of knowing and probably trusting the place, and its staff. Most larger hospices also have education centres, which we shall discuss in a later chapter.

In 1999, according to the National Council for Hospices and

Palliative Care Services, there were 172 adult hospices in England, Wales and Northern Ireland. There were 15 children's
hospices, and 3 AIDS units, making a total of 190.[9] In Scotland,
where a parallel organization, the Scottish Partnership Agency,
acts as a unifying body, there were 16 adult hospices, one children's hospice and one AIDS hospice.

What then is a hospice? The answer will vary in different
cultures and countries, and I can only write with any authority
about Britain. A hospice is a small specialist unit, in a free-
standing building or group of buildings, giving palliative care
to a limited number of people, mostly with some form of
cancer, both in the facility itself and in the wider community.
It typically has from 8 to 30 beds, one or more specialist
doctors, a relatively large number of nurses, a chaplain or two,
a social worker, and various paramedical staff some of whom
are part-time. The local community, lay and professional, sup-
ports it, and it is a place where the aim, not always achieved,
is that people should live until they die. It is friendly, welcoming and peaceful and there is an air of calm. It is a deeply
spiritual place. This series of descriptions mixes reality with
fantasy. Not every patient would recognize this as a description
of the new home that they have found, and few of the staff
would subscribe to it in its entirety.

It might be useful here to set out the Essentials of Hospice
Care as Bruce Rumbold summarizes them in his book *Help-
lessness and Hope*, based on his participant-research work in a
Manchester hospice.

1 Management by an experienced clinical team integrated
into the work of the whole medical community and giving
effective continuity of care.
2 Understanding control of the common symptoms of
terminal disease, especially pain in all its aspects, will
enable patients to live to their maximum potential, and will
at times herald unexpected remissions and/or the possibility of further active treatment.
3 Skilled and experienced team nursing which calls for
confident leadership by the ward sister and easy communication among its members.

4 A full interdisciplinary staff meeting frequently for discussion. The doctor does not relinquish his clinical responsibility but a member of another discipline may sometimes assume leadership for a particular patient or family.

5 A Home Care programme, active or consultative and involving all the relevant disciplines, must be developed according to local circumstances so that it can be integrated with the hospitals, the family practices of the area and its own beds.

6 Recognition of the patient and his family as the unit of care and of the family as part of the caring team. They may need support, not only in meeting physical demands but also in their own search for reality and meaning.

7 A mixed group of patients. Although the current in hospice care in the US is especially concerned with the 'dying cancer patient and his family', a good community is usually a mixed one, and hospices may include among their concerns those with long-term illness, chronic pain, and in some cases frailty and old age.

8 Bereavement follow-up to identify those who are especially vulnerable and to give support in co-operation with the family doctor and any local services which can be involved.

9 Methodical recording and analysis will monitor clinical practice and, co-ordinated with relevant research where possible, lead to soundly based practice and teaching.

10 Teaching in all aspects of terminal care. Special units should be a resource, stimulating initial interest, giving experience and passing on tested knowledge to others in both general and specialist fields.

11 Imaginative use of the architecture available. Many hospices will not be able to build anew and have to adapt a building in order to combine privacy with openness and community and a sense of home with efficient operation.

12 An efficient and approachable administration, essential to any field of human need and care, is here required to give security to patients, families and staff. Efficiency is both comforting and time saving. So far hospices have shown

that their operation is cost-effective as well as appropriate and humane.

13 A readiness for the cost of commitment and the search for meaning. Devotion has been an outstanding character-istic of past and present hospices. Willingness to face this demand has a fundamental bearing on the way the work is done and the stability of the staff. A Christian Hospice will be aware of the presence of the crucified and risen Christ in the midst.[10]

Rumbold did his research in the mid 1980s, and while his desiderata remain very helpful, more recent developments have complicated the issue of what a hospice is. The rise of palliative medicine as a separate discipline, and the formation of palliative care teams in hospitals, has led to the adoption of the description 'Specialist Palliative Care Unit' for hospice units, and some hospices have been tempted to change their names, while most have remembered that hospices are rec-ognized and loved charities. Some hospices, especially quite small ones, have difficulty fulfilling the description of special-ist units, and the National Council for Hospice and Specialist Palliative Care Services (for England, Wales and Northern Ireland), along with the Scottish Partnership Agency, are currently looking, yet again, at the question of definition.

Yet it might be true to say that all of us who work in the area assume that we know what a hospice is, and in the later chapters of this book I hope to be able to sift truth from illusion.

THE HOSPICE AS A RELIGIOUS INSTITUTION

This is certainly a common perception. When we look at the roots of St Christopher's and other similar foundations it is not surprising that those of the community who have paid attention to the hospice movement expect a religious and specifically Christian emphasis in care and general outlook. From time to time word reaches us of patients in the general hospital who feel they are not holy enough to come to the hospice and there are also, but less often, rumours of those who do not find it sufficiently catholic or evangelical! Senior Registrars on rotation in the two hospices and the various palliative care units in Edinburgh recently remarked that there is a different ethos in St Columba's, or that there is perceived to be, simply because of its name and because it has a chapel, centrally situated and well advertised. The Marie Curie Centres in Edinburgh and Glasgow have fairly recently appointed wholetime chaplains, but have as yet, no designated 'holy' space and are perceived to be more secular.

There are other perceptions of the hospice movement which may have a grain of truth in them, but may also be a species of urban myth. It has been argued that in order to find a place in a hospice, the patient must be articulate and able to argue with the doctor and put up a persuasive case. 'All your patients are middle-class,' is an assertion which is occasionally made and easily disproved by observation, as is the accusation that we only admit 'nice' people! A similar 'myth' is generated by all those who quite sincerely say that they have been struck by the atmosphere of peace and serenity as soon as they have crossed the hospice threshold. This is perhaps the real miracle of hospice care, because serenity can be projected even if the wards are short-staffed, the office staff are having a meeting about a grievance, and the chaplain has not even showed up. Those who work in hospices are ordinary people who are liable to weariness, depression, personality clashes, ambition and laziness, like anyone else.

Hospices have been criticized for using famous names and important people in their effort to raise money and public profile. A President with a title – preferably one that is hereditary – gives a certain status to a small and struggling organization. It is useful to have bankers, stockbrokers, businessmen, retired surgeons, lawyers and the like on the Board of Governors. Usually a clergyperson or two is there also and bishops are chosen as Patrons and thus the standing of the hospice is assured. It is equally true that it could be useful to have one's name connected with a hospice since the movement had such a strong popular appeal as a respectable charity. AIDS hospices may have much more difficulty in raising funds and acquiring famous patrons.

Critics of the modern hospice movement have often concen-
trated on its 'respectable and middle-class' image, with its
overtones of superiority to the mere NHS hospital, and insofar
as supporters of the hospice idea have denigrated the excellent work of the NHS, criticisms are well deserved. Hospices
are still basically respectable and middle-class. Why should
small, specialized units, where there is a high staff-patient
ratio, and very pleasant, well-maintained surroundings receive
so much public applause, and even public funding, when the
money raised by charity and from NHS resources could be
better deployed in improving hospital services?

In 1992 Colin Douglas, an Edinburgh geriatrician and novel-
ist, who has a wonderful way with words, wrote in his column
in the *British Medical Journal* a broadside against the hospice
movement which earned him hard words from its leaders.
The article encapsulates several objections to the hospice movement. 'Why should care at the end of an illness be so separate
from all that has gone before? Why should only the minority
who die of malignancies – and precious few even of them –
be singled out for deluxe dying? And why should a large
and general need be left to the scanty and scandalously
choosy efforts of a patchwork of local charities with one hand
in the coffers of the NHS and the other in the church bazaar
economy?' He does say later that 'in its time the hospice movement served several useful functions; as a brave new cause
when standards of terminal care were broadly lamentable; as
a base for the development of nursing skills and service inno-
vations such as home care for the dying; and as a first home
for that useful scientific, clinical and educational endeavour,
the specialty of palliative care.' 'Well done, thanks and goodbye,' he continues. 'The hospice movement – with all its
paraphernalia of flower arrangers, charity balls, committee
loads of duchesses and agreeable secluded little places to die
amid leafy glades – no longer has a useful role. It is now a
distraction from the main business of improving the every-
day care of the ordinary dying. The NHS should now take
charge . . . the more adaptable palliative care doctors will find
themselves welcome in the real world . . . why not a hospice
heritage trail?' [11]

No wonder there was anger among hospice staff. But the article neatly puts a finger on the dangers that surround such a 'prophetic' movement. There is uncontrolled adulation in some places – 'you are all angels!' The more praise there is, the less hospices are able to accept hostile criticism. The use of money received from public funds must be justified. Most people do not die in hospices, and general services require investment and improvement. But the time for the hospice heritage trail might be some distance away. The 'Lady Bountiful' image, if it was ever deserved, is being shed. The movement does give great scope for voluntary service in many departments. If at first it was those who could afford not to work who offered their services that is no longer true. More and more volunteers are being recruited from the families and friends of patients. Units are increasingly professionalized and there are few leafy glades left. They have mostly become the sites of education departments or car parks! Why should not the dying, even a minority of them, have the best in surroundings and total care? As specialist palliative care units and wards are set up in NHS hospitals, the need for hospices may diminish, but it is too early to write an obituary. Honest and well expressed criticism is necessary, or we will believe what our admirers tell us, and we can only be grateful to those who take the trouble to point out our faults.

Recently, in her book *The Dying Process*, Julia Lawton has written of her experiences as a researcher in a hospice which works within the National Health Service, and which was facing severe cutbacks and the attendant lowering of morale which these inevitably bring. She confesses her previous lack of immediate contact with death, and her assumption, shared by many, of a 'somewhat romanticised conception of dying patients resting comfortably in bed, mentally alert, calm and reassured',[12] which, as she rightly says, is all too prevalent in hospice-friendly literature. Not surprisingly the reality was painful. 'What I was unprepared for . . . was the visible signs of bodily decay; the stench of incontinence; the lethargy and despondency of patients, many of whom had struggled with their illness for months or years; and the burnout and exhaustion experienced by their families and friends.' It would unbalance this book to spend too long at this point discussing Lawton's experiences, which in many respects surprised me. In particular I have not been aware of the special hospice smell which she encountered: 'the odour of excreta, vomit and rotting flesh'.[13] 'I was, for example, always struck by the smell when I first walked into the building. It was not the typical antiseptic smell one would expect of a hospital setting; it was more pungent and more nauseating; a combination of essential oils such as lemon and cinnamon, interlaced with the odour of vomit and excreta . . . it was always there.'[14] Since this has only very occasionally been my experience I can only conclude that research was done at an unfortunate time in this hospice. I first heard of this work on a discussion programme on the BBC when one of the participants remarked that having learned about the research he would never let any of his relatives go to a hospice, and no wonder, if what she has written is generally true.

Nevertheless Lawton has very valid points to make, and it is good for hospice professionals to be challenged in their assumptions of public perceptions. She is particularly acute in her description of what she calls the 'sequestration of the unbounded body'.[15] Patients do get moved to side rooms to give other patients peace; they are sometimes sedated for the benefit of the relatives or the staff; there is such a thing as a social death, which can occur long before the body ceases to breathe. Honesty in facing the less pleasant features of the care of the dying, and the ability to renounce the rosy descriptions of hospices in some of our literature, are necessary, and anthropological and sociological research, which challenges the assumptions of hospice pioneers and the perceptions of the public is necessary and to be welcomed. Patients do lose the will to live, they are often bored, they can be impatient to die, and disappointed if they wake up in the morning. There are smells and waste matter, and not all procedures are pleasant. Yet the testimony of so many patients and families is that things could have been so much worse. They feel that they have been rescued and reassured, and the amount of support that hospices receive from grateful relatives cannot all stem from the guilt of those who let their loved ones be cared for by others.

CHAPLAINS IN HOSPICES

With such an evidently Christian origin, both in the Middle Ages and the middle twentieth century, it was only to be expected that chaplains would be among the first appointments when a new hospice opened. Chaplaincy in the general hospital has developed as a profession in the last few decades, and at first hospice chaplaincy could be seen as a subsection of general chaplaincy. But soon the differences became apparent. A hospital chaplain might be responsible for a unit of 500 or more patients and a corresponding number of staff. She would relate to the NHS as well as to her church, and to the hospital management. The hospice chaplain might be wholetime and have a mere thirty patients and around one hundred staff in her 'parish'. 'So,' asked a critical colleague not unkindly, 'what do you find to do all day?' That certainly is a sensitive question. The answer has something to do with intensity, with constant crisis, and with specialization. While more and more patients spend very short times in hospital, patients in hospices return several times with short intervals at home, or come in for continuing care. Families are very much in evidence and often need as much counsel as the patients. Staff are under particular strains. What could be seen as favouring a small privileged group might become a paradigm for wider application.

Two contrary forces appear to be at work. On the one hand there is a growing perception of the need for spiritual care for patients with very serious illness, and for their carers. On the other, spirituality is in danger of being taken from the 'religious' sphere, and made a much more general concept, delivered by a variety of staff members, some of whom might be chaplains. Since the 1960s the process of secularization has proceeded apace in the UK. Statistics appear to show that fewer people regularly attend mainstream churches, and indeed that specifically religious matters affect fewer folk.[16] Therefore chaplaincy is in danger of becoming marginalized, if not treated as an interesting relic from the old days, tolerated in hospices because of their origins. Later I will look more closely at the concept of spirituality. Meanwhile the growing number of hospices which appoint wholetime chaplains, or co-operate with hospitals in shared chaplaincy, might seem to indicate that the place of the chaplain is not so threatened as we sometimes fear.

SUPPORT FOR CHAPLAINS

Since hospice chaplaincy was a new branch of the profession of hospital chaplaincy, it was necessary for support mechanisms to be set up for the small but growing number of new appointments. I was for several years the only hospice chaplain in Scotland, and I am grateful for the support of the hospital chaplains in these years of isolation and after. Meetings about spiritual care in hospices were called by concerned chaplains at Birmingham and St Giles Hospice, Lichfield, and after a consultation at St George's House, Windsor, in 1985, at length an Association of Hospice Chaplains came into being, which has held an annual Conference, usually at All Saints, London Colney. This has given a forum for learning, and sharing information and knowledge. Members of the Executive have also been able to represent hospice chaplaincy in the counsels of the College of Health Care Chaplains and in national bodies concerned with palliative care. Both wholetime and part-time chaplains have benefited from the Association, and many of us have continued our membership of national chaplaincy bodies.

To be able to meet with and talk to those in the same field has been invaluable for us. The association has also been able to put hospice chaplaincy into profitable dialogue with churches and government. It has held together the rapidly changing group of chaplains in hospices, and given us a reference point and a voice.

FOR FURTHER THOUGHT

1 Are chaplains necessary in hospices?
2 Do hospices reflect the society in which they have developed?

NOTES

1 Lawrence Stone, *The Family, Sex and Marriage in England 1500–1800*. Harmondsworth: Penguin, abridged edition 1979, p. 57.

2 Membership Book of George Street Baptist Church, Glasgow.
3 David Rorie, 'Hastening the death of the aged, infirm and sick', in *British Medical Journal* (1933) II, pp. 611–12; reprinted in *Folk Medicine and Folk Tradition in Scotland: the Writings of David Rorie*, ed. David Buchan. Edinburgh: Canongate Academic 1994.
4 G. Gorer, 'The pornography of death' in *Encounter* (October 1955).
5 For many further details of the early development of homes for the dying see Clare Humphreys, 'The establishment of the first hospices in England' in *Mortality* 6:2 (July 2001).
6 D. Clark, 'Originating a movement' in *Mortality* 3:1, p. 45.
7 *Ibid.*, p. 50.
8 David Farrant, *A History of St Barnabas' Hospice*. Worthing 1999.
9 National Council for Hospice and Specialist Palliative Care, *Briefing 1*. October 1999.
10 Bruce D. Rumbold, *Helplessness and Hope: Pastoral Care in Terminal Illness*. London: SCM Press 1986, pp. 100–1.
11 Colin Douglas in *British Medical Journal* 304 (29 February 1992), p. 579.
12 Julia Lawton, *The Dying Process: Patients' Experiences of Palliative Care*. London: Routledge 2000, p. vii.
13 *Ibid.*, p. 135.
14 *Ibid.*, p. 77.
15 *Ibid.*, pp. 122ff.
16 See, for example, Peter Brierley, *The Tide Is Running Out: What the English Church Attendance Survey Reveals*. London: Christian Research 2000.

CHAPTER TWO

Living with Death and Dying

I have worked now for more than twenty years in a hospice. During that time I have become aware of the many facets that there are to the study of the dying process and of death itself, and of how much change there has been in the human perception of death, particularly in the last two hundred years. For good reasons, within the Western world, death has become pre-eminently the concern of the medical and nursing professions. Just as most births in Britain now take place in hospital, so do most deaths. This is such a commonplace that it seems to many people only right and natural to die in a hospital ward or a hospice room, cared for by professionals, with the family indeed there, but not as principal actors in the scene. Modern houses are said not to be well adapted to nursing the very sick, with small rooms, narrow staircases, and toilets on a different level from the living space. Yet from all accounts most people in Britain, at least until the Second World War, lived in much more cramped and insanitary conditions than would be tolerated today.

Certainly today there is much more movement of population than in previous generations, and the extended family is far more scattered for most people. This extension of course depends on perception. Elderly women might complain that the family has moved to the other side of the city, or that all the children are in New Zealand! Even if the family is near, it is very likely that those who would formerly have been the natural carers are working outside the home, and unable or unwilling to accept the burden of nursing a dying parent. Economic circumstances have dictated a different pattern of care. People also expect more intensive care from doctors and nurses, and physical discomfort which continues for any time is seen to be a failure on their part. Higher expectations have led to greater efforts, and the threat of litigation when treatment fails lurks in the background of medical minds.

It is also possible to see a quite altered attitude to death in Western society in these last decades. The changing approaches to death in different civilizations and periods of history make a fascinating and illuminating study, so long as we remember that not everyone at a given time has the same outlook. Even in as small a group of islands as Britain, there are communities which still retain older traditions of care and of mourning, and these are not all in remote places. Very traditional religious groups and ethnic communities would not fit easy generalizations. Opposition to cremation, for example, is still fierce among the Free and Free Presbyterian Churches of Scotland, to the extent that there is still no crematorium in Inverness. In England the question is scarcely even argued among Strict Baptists. Burial is the only right way for these traditional Christians, and although the Roman Catholic Church some years ago lifted its ban on cremation, many Catholics would still prefer to be buried. Other communities within the British Isles have retained customs worthy of our study, although it is naive to think that we can easily reincorporate lost rites into modern urban society.[1] It is impossible to go backwards and rediscover a lost history. We are bound to our present, and must live fruitfully in it.

HUMAN RESPONSE TO DEATH

To understand the appeal of the hospice movement, it is relevant to examine briefly the history of human response to death, at least within certain limits, beginning with the Middle Ages in the West. 'No other epoch has laid so much stress as the expiring Middle Ages on the thought of death,' wrote Johan Huizinga. 'An everlasting call of *memento mori* resounds through life . . . since the thirteenth century, the popular preaching of the mendicant orders had made the eternal admonition to remember death swell into a sombre chorus ringing throughout the world.'[2] He goes on to describe vividly the Dance of Death, and the ever-present icons of mortality that confronted Western European people in the centuries before the Reformation.

Although the work of Philippe Ariès has been criticized for taking too narrow a view of the literature and geography of dying, his great book, *The Hour of Our Death*, first published in English translation in 1981, remains a source of both information and pleasure. He began by studying the history of the large urban cemeteries in France and was impressed by the changes which have become evident in the last two hundred years. In the Middle Ages he found 'the narrowness and anonymity of the graves, the piling up of bodies, the reuse of graves, the storing of bones in charnels'[3] to be evidence of indifference toward the dead. 'Christianity had disposed of the dead by abandoning them to the Church where they were forgotten.' Only in the late eighteenth century was there detected a new sensibility which 'rejected the traditional indifference and a piety was invented that became so popular and so widespread in the romantic era that it was believed to have existed from the beginning of time'.[4] As his investigations of tombs, cemeteries, writings and wills progressed he modified his scheme, and in his book, he divides attitudes into three huge sections. The first he calls the tame death, expected and accepted, which was the pattern until the Renaissance. Then there was the age of remote and imminent death, death untamed, which led to a concentration on the lessons of dying, and on making 'a good death'. In the Romantic era of the eighteenth century he quotes from poetry, novels and journals to illustrate the 'Beautiful Death' of romantic heroes and heroines and wonderful literature of consolation. In the modern and contemporary world he finds the Invisible Death – death denied. Here he writes of the transfer of the place of death to the hospital, the discreet funeral, the medicalization of all the processes of death and grief and the demand for dignity in dying. He refers very briefly to the new idea, or the old one revived, of the hospice. It is impossible in a few words to do justice to the magnificent sweep and the detailed descriptions of this book. Ariès has at least established a pattern of change that has deeply affected our society. Alongside Ariès we can listen to Ernest Becker, who 'taught us that awe, fear and ontological anxiety were natural accompaniments to our contemplation of the fact of death'.[5] Human fascination with death has produced great literature, great heroism and not a little dread. Religious changes have signalled the most obvious changes of attitudes over the years.

Clearly, in those countries where it took root, the sixteenth-century Reformation changed attitudes to death. The Reformers quite soon disposed of the idea of prayers for the dead, masses for the departed, and the idea of purgatory. Death became the moment after which no choice was possible, and while it remained terrible, it was also rediscovered as the gateway to eternal life. 'The faithful in Christian England were conditioned to expect a happier life beyond the painful passages of dying, on the other side of this present vale of tears. For catholics, eternal bliss came after the pains of purgatory; for protestants, the passage of the soul to heaven could take place in an instant so long as it belonged to one of the elect. It is hard to judge which religion allowed the greatest degree of equanimity.'[6]

It is interesting to remember the explicitly medieval roots of hospices as conceived by Dame Cicely Saunders. There has been an attempt to return to a view of death which accepts its inevitability and asserts its rightness in the scheme of creation. We have been given permission by studies and teaching from Elisabeth Kübler-Ross onwards to practise the art of dying gracefully. But to understand the present situation it is necessary to trace the story of our arrival here. People have not always regarded death in the way that we do.

In *The Revival of Death* Tony Walter writes:

for millennia, death has disrupted communities and the language of death has been the communal language of religion. In the modern era, however, the human encounter with death has been split – on the one hand into expert medical discourse and associated bureaucratic procedures, and on the other hand into an intensely personal sense of loss . . . The Age of Reason shifted death from the frame of

religion into the frame of reason, from the frame of sin and
fate to the frame of statistical probability.[7]

Religion is still closely connected with death, even if it is
only acknowledged by the presence of a minister at the
funeral, and the singing of hymns. Hospice experience is that
the chaplain is seen as a useful person to have around when
someone dies. The intense attention to rites and ceremonies
which characterized at least the wealthier parts of society
until very recently has given way to professionally well managed preparation of the body and funeral services, in which
the chaplain plays a significant part, sometimes more as a
friend and companion than as a religious official.

CHRISTIAN BELIEFS ABOUT DEATH AND DYING

At the beginning of a new millennium it is important to
examine current beliefs about the meaning of death and its
aftermath. In a secular age when public religious observance,
at least among Christians, seems to be on the wane, what may
a chaplain assume about the people for whom she cares? In a
congregation she might expect some uniformity of belief, in
salvation, resurrection and the purpose of God. She would of
course be mistaken, for regular worshippers and financial
supporters of the institutional church have as varied views
and experiences as the rest of the population. But at least, in
a particular congregation, there might be some words and
ideas held in common, and certain liturgical texts, such as
hymns, understood and shared. Church members are wary
of letting the pastor know too much of their individual and
private theologies, at least until a great deal of trust is built up,
but there must be assumed an adherence to certain norms of
belief and action.

Among those of the general population who find their
way into a hospice, and are willing to speak and listen to the
chaplain, there will be a far wider spectrum of beliefs and
unbeliefs, and there will be less inhibition on expressing them.
Indeed they can be expressed with great vehemence. 'I will
not go to any heaven without dogs,' stated an argumentative

patient with perfect seriousness. It would not have been wise to point out that most biblical references to dogs are fairly pejorative!

In his book *The Eclipse of Eternity*, Tony Walter begins his 'sociology of the afterlife' by referring to the medieval Hôtel Dieu de Beaune in Burgundy. At the end of the one ward is an altarpiece of the last Judgement, with Christ seated in glory, and an archangel weighing the souls of the deceased. On his left the damned descend to hell; on his right the saved ascend to glory. There was no escape from the statement of faith. Only two modern British hospice logos out of one hundred and thirty confidently affirm that death is not the end, and 'none as much as hint that there could be a choice of post-mortem destinations'.[8] He claims, with much justification, that 'until the late nineteenth century for Protestants and until the nineteen-sixties for Catholics our fate in the hereafter has been central for Christianity.' There is in fact great confusion on the subject. If a new catechism is produced that is not clear about hell, or if a church leader denounces the doctrine of eternal punishment, there is an outcry in the press that traditional morality is in danger, but if a conservative church firmly proclaims the dangers of hell fire, then there is another outcry, this time about outworn and dangerous beliefs.

When an American Baptist group distributed copied of Jonathan Edwards's graphic eighteenth-century sermon *Sinners in the Hands of an Angry God* to households in a housing estate in Edinburgh I was confronted with angry members of our staff and accused (since I am a Baptist even if of a slightly less abrasive sort) of frightening old ladies! It seems that the old belief that fear of hell kept folk in order dies hard. Two articles by a hospital chaplain[9] recently published in an American hospice journal on 'Spiritual Terrorism' and 'Spiritual Abuse' indicate that at least in the US the fear of hell and punishment is still alive and well.

In the high Middle Ages we may reasonably assume that only a very few brave spirits challenged the belief in the eternal punishment of the wicked. In our present situation the experience of chaplains is that only a tiny minority of dying people even contemplates being afraid of hell, although there may be more fear experienced than is expressed. This makes for a fascinating intellectual journey. Great changes in expectation have occurred in the last few hundred years.

It was the Reformation which allowed, despite the intentions of Luther and Calvin, a new questioning process. In the seventeenth century a number of adventurous thinkers in the Commonwealth period in England began to challenge Protestant orthodoxy on the subjects of the Trinity and eternal torment, and some of these early Socinians and Arians questioned the compatibility of a God of love and eternal punishment.[10] Nevertheless the confessions of the Church continued to teach the parting of the ways after death.

In the nineteenth century teachers both in the Church of England and among the Nonconformists challenged the older doctrines and proclaimed 'The Larger Hope'. Conservatives like the Baptist C. H. Spurgeon seized on such teaching, which included both Universalists who believed in the ultimate salvation of all people, and proponents of conditional immortality, who believed in the annihilation of the wicked, as signs of the 'downgrade of true religion' and continued vigorously to proclaim eternal punishment of the wicked. Gradually such teaching became confined to written creeds and to a minority of evangelical teachers, and sermons on hell fire passed out of the preacher's repertoire. The injustice of never-ending punishment, the greater stress on the love of God and the diminished certainty of believers led to the dissolution of the old themes. Outside the Church, Western society simply ignored such abstruse ideas. If there is a hell it is here and now. Even the terrible events of the twentieth century have not led to a revival of hell as a popular theological doctrine. As David Lodge remarked of his newly enlightened Catholics, in his novel *How Far Can You Go?*, 'at some point in the 1960s Hell disappeared . . . by Hell we mean of course the traditional Hell of Roman Catholics, a place where you would burn for all eternity if you were unlucky enough to die in a state of mortal sin.'[11] What had happened amongst all but the most conservative Protestants some decades before had now spread much farther.

A fascinating account of the changes in English attitudes to death is given in Pat Jalland's book *Death in the Victorian Family*.[12] Using the letters and papers mainly of well-to-do families, she charts the change of attitudes from an open and warm Christianity, which felt no difficulty in talking about death and the afterlife in letters of consolation and inscriptions on tombstones, to a much more restrained and secular expression of grief and sympathy. Victorian agnosticism, falling rates of mortality and the trauma of the Great War all had their effect.

Jalland shows that Christians were sustained by a system of belief in life after death which was reflected in memoirs, poetry and hymns and which gave a shape to mourning and grief, whereas agnostics lacked a substitute for Christian rituals of death and mourning. 'Deathbeds for agnostics entirely lacked the consolations of the good Christian death, and their accounts were chiefly notable for their brevity.'[13] This led to great isolation in bereavement – 'a solitude beyond the reach of God or man'. Yet the Victorian agnostic may still have had Christian family and friends to give some meaning to his experience. Jalland comments that in the twentieth century people also have no belief in 'a positive view of death, but without the cultural context of the Victorian agnostics, surrounded as they were by Christians for whom death was an essential and familiar part of their life and faith. Without a dominant Christianity against which to define unbelief, the meaning of death has largely been excluded from public culture, except for the inherited rituals of the burial or cremation service. But the loss of the meaning of death has also been a loss in the meaning of human life, a cultural problem which post-Christian societies are still trying to resolve.'[14]

Jalland also spells out the effect that the great number of deaths of soldiers in the First World War had on rituals and beliefs. No longer could there be adequate burial and mourning rituals when so many soldiers were killed in such a short period. She quotes Jay Winter as saying that 'the individuality of death was buried under literally millions of corpses'.[15] It was hard for families to believe that their sons had died when there was no corpse to view, and the flourishing of spiritualism and the incidence of unresolved grief can be explained by the idea that dead soldiers somehow survived and deserved to be in heaven. It was in these conditions that the equation of death for one's country with martyrdom was made. John Buchan wryly claims this in his ballad 'Fisher Jamie':

> And noo he's in a happier land –
> It's Gospel truth and Gospel law
> That Heaven's yett[16] maun open stand
> To folk that for their country fa'.[17]

The stern-sounding beliefs of earlier centuries have broken down in our times, and been succeeded by a mixture of dogmatic doubt and vague yearnings. It seems to be assumed that God is obliged 'by Gospel truth and Gospel law' to accept everyone of goodwill and that the old doctrines of salvation and resurrection are relics of a past age. Far from people being terrified to die because of fear of what awaits them they often express a great confidence in a better time coming, and their fears are much more immediate. They express fear of dying, not of death itself.

Walter has argued that there may be nothing very new about the agnosticism with which most people regard death. He points out that it is difficult to discover what ordinary folk thought, as what is written is in the domain of clergy, who have had a vested interest in keeping the traditional Christian belief alive. He adduces examples from Brittany and Ireland that popular tales were told outside the control of the priests, well into modern times, and that this could well have been the norm in Europe in previous centuries.[18] I can recall being startled when a church member whose husband had recently died remarked to me that it was strange that he, a non-church member, believed in life after death. 'I don't,' she said. 'After all, no one has come back to tell us.'

RITUALS AND STORIES

Rituals have been and still are important. Actual belief-systems are much harder to pinpoint. Opinion polls of various kinds have in recent years shown that belief in God and in the afterlife are still quite prevalent despite the rapid fall in church-going.[19] Experience in the hospice has shown that the chaplain can neither rely on nor ignore popular beliefs about what happens at death and thereafter. Death is a great mystery, whether it is considered in a theological volume, or experienced by a hard-bitten post-modern woman. And it remains a mystery to those of us whose calling it is to tend and watch over the dying.

Certainly death is an interesting subject. The number of books, journals and articles devoted to it proves that. Newspaper features, and television and radio programmes portray it in various guises. At a time when images of violent death, in wars as in former Yugoslavia, in acts of terrorism such as the destruction of the World Trade Centre in New York or in natural disasters as in Mozambique seemingly make sudden and unnatural death a matter of little consequence, the death of a child in a road accident in our village, or the death by apparent neglect of a resident in a nursing home, arouse public interest and anger. On the one hand we watch death in far off places, and have to make ourselves callous, or we would be in constant mourning; on the other we are still capable of being deeply moved by the unfairness of death. Several writers and journalists have recently published accounts of their own encounter with cancer, leading in most cases to premature death. There is a great appetite for death stories.

An interesting recent book, *The Place of the Dead*,[20] contains essays on themes of death and remembrance in late-medieval and early modern Europe, and illustrates how many attitudes were possible, and also how little in some ways things have changed. Will-making is still important; the place of burial, the re-use of graves, the possibility of ghosts and revenants, themes of judgement and punishment, all areas covered by the contributors, still are of relevance. Yet of course there have been great societal changes. We are not the same as our early modern ancestors. We know far more about the human body, and about the workings of the mind. We no longer have recognized rituals to deal with the fear and uncertainty caused by the transition of death. As Norbert Elias says in an essay on 'The Loneliness of the Dying':

In the presence of dying people – and of mourners – we therefore see with particular clarity a dilemma characteristic of the present stage of the civilizing process. A shift towards informality has caused a whole series of traditional patterns of behaviour in great crisis-situations of human life, including the use of ritual phrases, to become suspect and embarrassing for many people. The task of finding the right word and the right gesture therefore falls back on the individual . . . it is only the institutionalized routines of hospitals that give a social framework to the situation of dying. These, however, are mostly devoid of feeling, and contribute much to the isolation of the dying.[21]

Elias neatly pinpoints one of the ways in which death in Western society differs from death in most previous eras. It has become individualized. You have to do it on your own. There are no ritual norms any more. Hospices can at least give a context of shared experience and can promote communication between the dying person and her family and carers.

Despite the privatization of death, it remains firmly in the centre of human experience. It can be argued that we have become more sensitive to its terrors and more able to counsel the dying and the bereaved at the same time as death has left home and disappeared into hospitals. Society is now aware of the hurt that the death of a parent inflicts on a young child, and there are self-help organizations and counselling available for all concerned.

I was sharply reminded of this when recently I visited the grave of my mother on the sixtieth anniversary of her death. She died unexpectedly a few days before I was due to start school and I have few memories of her. But I can vividly remember how I was told of her death by the shocked family friend with whom I was living during my mother's time in hospital for a routine operation. I can remember my father crying and thinking how strange this was, but I certainly do not remember anyone trying to explain what had happened or being aware of what was happening to a child at a sensitive time. The new experience of school, and the acquisition of a stepmother no doubt took up my attention. But the scars remain, and from time to time I go in search of my mother, by talking to the increasingly elderly people who remember her, by trying to answer the questions of my own children, by seeking out her cousins and more distant members of her family. But sometimes grief can ambush me, as it did when I visited the cemetery with flowers.

I am comforted to think that today I would have had a skilled counsellor, and that support systems would be in place if I needed them. Parents often do not have confidence to speak to their children if someone very close is dying. A professional who is outside the family may often be the best person to take on that task. Schools are more aware of the need for pastoral care of pupils, and most people are willing to accept help when death comes close. The relatively new custom of making shrines at the scene of a road accident is worth noting. It seems that by laying flowers, school scarves, furry toys and other objects at the roadside young people are able to express their grief in an acceptable way.

THE POWER OF THE DEAD

Perhaps one of the reasons that hospices and the care of the dying have so caught public imagination is that there is still an inherent, implicit belief in the continuing influence and even power of the dead. Superstition is by no means extinct, and the absolute division between the living and the dead is still questioned. Thomas Kselman, writing of nineteenth-century Brittany, records the conviction that 'for a certain period after their death, the dead continue to lead a life that resembles our own. They return to the places they frequented when alive, sometimes to harm the living. The dead wandered along the roads in the neighbourhood and went back to their houses, but they were especially likely to inhabit the local cemetery and were sensitive to any insult they may suffer from the living. The dead were known to visit the living, especially at night. Women were advised not to sweep after sunset so as to avoid brushing out of doors the dead who had returned home.'[22] What is described as being the case in nineteenth-century France could be replicated in many societies throughout the world. In Greenock in the 1950s all Catholic households covered every reflective surface in the house while an occupied coffin lay in it, and so did many Protestants, lest the departed soul should see itself and be disturbed. This is folk religion, and we may consider that it is entirely out-moded in our post-Christian society. But it might equally be argued that New Age ideas, the rise of modern paganism and similar beliefs, and lingering suspicion of death all point to the possibility that many otherwise enlightened people have very ambivalent feelings about the dead. The 'restless dead' are well documented in Keith Thomas's *Religion and the Decline of Magic*[23] and in Ariès' *The Hour of Our Death*.[24]

The control of the dead over the living is exerted in many subtle ways. Possibly not many are frightened by the possi-bility of reappearance, but the wishes of the deceased can have a strong effect on the living. There are those who have not remarried because to do so would be to flout the expressed wish of the deceased spouse. There are unmarried daughters who have remained so because of what father said. Spoken or even written instructions from the dead can have a lasting effect on the living. 'I am my sister's living representative on earth and I am determined to raise enough money to buy a scanner for the hospital.' For Susan, whose sister died in her thirties in the hospice, this is a task to be pursued with reli-gious zeal. There are numerous small charities started by the dead, whether organizations devoted to suppressing drunk driving or to a more obviously creative and positive task. Cicely Saunders began St Christopher's partly in memory of her Polish friend who gave her a first donation before he died.

Another way in which the dead can control the living is through wills. Futures are controlled and quarrels engendered and prolonged in families and beyond because of provisions and codicils. If the dying can threaten the healthy by con-stantly changing wills, then the dead can keep control by what they have laid down. Even by straightforward requests about funerals they can spread guilt when the provisions are overlooked or cannot be fulfilled. University departments of medicine do not necessarily accept all the bodies willed for research, and if they refuse, and the deceased has made his desires very clear, then the family may suffer acute guilt.

Wills can also tie future generations, with reversionary clauses and rights of life-rent, with provisions for the education of the grandchildren – I remember a student who had been left money on condition that he trained for the ministry – and bursaries for the education of those who fit the conditions of place of birth or family circumstances.

Spiritualism as a whole is too big a subject to be entered here, but it must be noted that there can be quite overt attempts to influence action and belief through apparent direct contact with the dead. If religion is defined as a search for truth, for a sign of the other, the divine, then seeking contact with the departed can be seen as a religious action. In the context of spiritualist churches it is as explicit as singing a hymn or praying. But unbelievers also go on this route to reassure themselves when someone they love dies. If it is true, as David Martin wrote in 1967,[25] that 10% of atheists believe in life after death, how many more wistful half-believers and agnostics may do so, and how many have dabbled, to use a pejorative word, in attempts to reach the dead. The dead can be in control of beliefs.

While hell fire preaching has suffered a decline, fear of judgement still exercises some social control, and the hope of gaining heaven can spur on to good works. But it is much less obvious and much more diffuse ways that the dead still influence the living and have power over otherwise sceptical people.

FOR FURTHER THOUGHT

1 Are we really sophisticated when we consider death and dying, or do we still carry with us older patterns of belief and feeling?

2 Can death ever be 'tamed'?

NOTES

1 See (among many other writings) Roger Grainger, 'Let death be death: lessons from the Irish wake' in *Mortality* 3:2, pp. 129–42, and David Ribner, 'A note on the Hassidic observance of the *Yahrzeit* custom and its place in the mourning process' in *ibid.* pp. 173–80.

2 J. Huizinga, *The Waning of the Middle Ages*. Harmondsworth: Penguin 1955, pp. 141–2.
3 Philippe Ariès, *The Hour of Our Death*. Harmondsworth: Penguin 1983, p. xi.
4 *Ibid.*
5 Ernest Becker, *The Denial of Death*. New York: Free Press 1997, p. xii.
6 David Cressy, *Birth, Death and Marriage: Ritual, Religion, and the Life-cycle in Tudor and Stuart England*. Oxford: Oxford University Press 1997, p. 383.
7 Tony Walter, *The Revival of Death*. London: Routledge 1994, p. 9.
8 Tony Walter, *The Eclipse of Eternity: a Sociology of the Afterlife*. Basingstoke: Macmillan 1996, p. 1.
9 B. C. Purcell in *American Journal of Hospice and Palliative Care* (May/June and July/August 1998).
10 See D. P. Walker, *The Decline of Hell: Seventeenth-century Discussions of Eternal Torment*. London: Routledge 1964.
11 David Lodge, *How Far Can You Go?* London: Secker & Warburg 1980, p. 113.
12 P. Jalland, *Death in the Victorian Family*. Oxford: Oxford University Press 1996.
13 *Op. cit.*, p. 357.
14 *Ibid.*
15 *Op. cit.*, p. 373.
16 Yett = gate.
17 John Buchan, 'Fisher Jamie', in W. H. Hamilton (ed.) *Holyrood: A Garland of Modern Scots Poems*. London: Dent.
18 Tony Walter, *The Eclipse of Eternity*, p. 54.
19 See, for one example, Tony Walter, *The Eclipse of Eternity*, p. 47.
20 Bruce Gordon and Peter Marshall, eds., *The Place of the Dead in Late Medieval and Early Modern Europe*. Cambridge: Cambridge University Press 2000.
21 Norbert Elias, *On Civilization, Power and Knowledge*. Chicago: University of Chicago Press 1988, p. 108.
22 Thomas Kselman, *Death and the Afterlife in Modern France*. Princeton, NJ: Princeton University Press, 1993, pp. 58–9.
23 Keith Thomas, *Religion and the Decline of Magic*. London: Weidenfeld and Nicolson 1971, chapter 19.
24 Philippe Ariès, *The Hour of Our Death*, pp. 396–400.
25 David Martin, *A Sociology of English Religion*. London: SCM Press 1967, p. 55.

CHAPTER THREE

The Hospice as Church

Since the hospice movement has such overtly religious origins, there are many aspects of its ethos which may make it possible for the healing, caring, loving institution to be perceived as a church in some sense, even when it has become secularized. Because hospices are managed in various ways it might even be possible to differentiate between those under central (e.g. Presbyterian or Episcopal) control and those which are independent yet adhering to the same principles (Congregationalist). Certainly chaplains and others are aware of the danger of the hospice becoming an alternative church, where an individual or even a family can obtain religious ordinances such as funerals without corresponding liability to any sort of church discipline. If the hospice maintains Sunday worship, then a person might choose to attend occasionally rather than become involved in a local church and thus avoid commitment. This is a temptation for an institution, especially for one which carries with it connotations of holiness and of a religious atmosphere, as many hospices rightly or wrongly are seen to do. The Sunday volunteer shares communion in the hospice chapel, and that is commendable and right. But should he do that rather than attend his own congregation? According to Shirley du Boulay, Dame Cicely Saunders regards St Christopher's Hospice chapel as her parish church.[1] The staff nurse chooses to work on Sunday mornings, and finds escort duty at the hospice chapel more congenial than going to her local church. How can that be at the same time accepted and discouraged?

Let us look at a hypothetical hospice, St James, in Anytown.

In the early 1970s a local committee, made up mainly from practising Anglicans, has been called into being by a forceful retired nurse, one of those charismatic characters that are required to get a hospice started. She is a devout Anglo-Catholic, who has caught the vision from Dame Cicely. She has read her books and articles, attended her lectures, and worked for a short time at St Christopher's. Her friends from the nursing, medical and church worlds mostly share her religious convictions, but they are of course quite willing to receive financial contributions from any source, church or not, for the work. Patrons are chosen, committees are set up, funds are raised, the property is bought, prayer meetings are held, and also fêtes and sales of work, and at last the hospice is ready to receive its first patient. But who will be the holy person? Who will embody the Christian ideal and be the public face of the faith of the founders? Who indeed will administer the Eucharist to this first patient? Will she want such ministration? The Vicar of the parish is hard pressed, and not quite in sympathy with the founder's ecclesiastical ideals. The local Nonconformist clergy are willing but puzzled and diffident. At length a suitable person is found. She is a married priest, looking for part-time work, and she formerly trained as a nurse. She seems ideal, and the Bishop agrees.

There is a service of inauguration, in which the Anglican Bishop, the Roman Catholic Bishop, the Moderator of the Province of the United Reformed Church and the Chairman of the Methodist District happily take part. The chapel is duly consecrated for all kinds of Christian worship. The Matron reads the Lessons and the Medical Director prays with eloquence, and it is all reported, with photographs, in the local press. All seems well – but the first patient is a Strict Baptist who not only does not want Anglican fripperies, but also says so loudly, and the second is a devout Sunni Muslim. Then there is the man who is a member of the British Humanist Association, and a whole host of patients who have not been in any church for years. Who is going to share in the Eucharist that the Governors have decreed must be celebrated each Sunday? Who will comfort the unbelieving? How will the hospice accommodate the unrepentant Nonconformist? It is here that we begin to encounter the secularized and diverse world in which the hospice must operate. If we hope that somehow in the holy atmosphere of a place caring for the dying we will reverse the tide of secularization, or if we believe that we are missionaries on that last boundary and that we are somehow immune to the increasingly prevalent rejection of the traditional life of the churches, then we are mistaken, and any attempt at chaplaincy which is trapped in such categories is doomed to irrelevancy at best.

Certainly the hospice must be seen within the context of the local manifestations of the Christian Church. In chaplaincy job descriptions there may well be a clause concerning the importance of the chaplain being in good standing with her church and the task of maintaining good relations with local clergy and churches. In many hospices, especially smaller units, the local clergy provide chaplaincy cover, possibly on a rota basis, and some measure of integration into the local community takes place. As hospices grow in confidence and financial security, salaried appointments to chaplaincy are made, part-time and increasingly wholetime, and this may lead to a distancing from the local churches. The best-qualified woman for the job may be working in a parish across the town, and the wholetime chaplain may live a distance from the unit. It is a common complaint of chaplains in health care that they are regarded with suspicion or neglect by their denominations, as those who have opted out of the 'real' ministry in the parish, or as subversives, too much interested in counselling and not interested or committed enough in proper church concerns. I hope the days are gone when clergy are offered hospital or hospice appointments because they find the daily life of a parish too strenuous, or because they have somehow 'failed' in other ministry. Hospice chaplaincy is not equivalent to semi-retirement! But all the churches need to assess how they are perceived to treat those who enter this field. If present conditions continue there is a real danger that health care chaplaincy will become a separate profession and that hospice chaplaincy, and especially wholetime chaplaincy, becomes a particular form of that profession. It is natural for those who face the same problems and share the

same insights to gather together for strength and support, but
it would be detrimental to the church at large if what we do
and learn is not integrated into the total vision.

WHAT IS A HOSPICE CHAPLAIN?

Hospices are intended to be places of interprofessional teamwork and trust. One of the main arguments in favour of
salaried appointments for chaplains is that the doctors, nurses and the others will then treat them as fellow professionals.
For many clergy, this is almost a new concept. Professionalism
is what they have been taught to avoid, at least under that
name. Vocation, calling, sacrifice, devotion to the faith, were
acceptable descriptions of the motives that led to the desire
for ordination. Professionalism suggested interest in status,
working to a contract, and agitation for better pay and conditions, rather than the setting of goals and standards, and the
pursuit of excellence. These harsh distinctions have not survived the modern changes in society, and the hospice, with
its idealistic origins, may be a good place for the concepts of
professionalism and vocation to come together and interact
fruitfully. Certainly many clergy have been accustomed to
work alone, whether by choice or necessity, and in a hospice
team the chaplain learns to be part of an information and
skill sharing group, working for the welfare of the patient. In
such a team she may find for the first time that she is valued
for her abilities and special accomplishments, and not only
for her office.

Is it then necessary to find a place in the life of the local
church? For the chaplain's own spiritual health, and for the
benefit of the church, I believe it is. Even when the denominational machinery seems to be isolating us, we need to remind
the hierarchy of our existence and importance, and we need
to be secure enough in our vocation and our professionalism
to offer whatever we can to the structures and communities
of our churches. We also need to worship and to continue to
learn and grow in our Christian pilgrimage along with the
whole variety of others whom we meet in the local church.

All this has been written on the assumption that the hospice has appointed a Christian chaplain or chaplains, in complete agreement with bishops, presbyteries and other authorities. But this, in the divided state of our churches, is not always easy to accomplish. Hospices are rightly jealous of their independence in choosing staff in all departments. They can be resentful if a chaplain simply arrives with a warrant from a church body. This can lead to misunderstandings that require much negotiation. Bishops may assume that they should appoint the local incumbent, and the hospice may think he is not suitable. But the bishop is short of priests, and is used to appointing clergy to the hospitals in their parishes. Why should the new hospice be different? There are plenty of disaster stories, especially about part-time denominational appointments. Sometimes the responsibility for the care of hospice patients of a particular denomination can be seen as just another parish chore, low on the list of priorities. Sometimes a minister can find visiting a hospice distasteful or frightening and that fear can present itself as aggression and a refusal to co-operate with other chaplains and staff. For some the very idea of interdisciplinary work is too new or dangerous to contemplate. It seems obvious, but it needs to be said – ordination does not convey an ability to care for very sick people and their families. And why should we expect it to do so?

With tact and patience on the part of the hospice management, and adaptability on the part of church authorities, good arrangements can usually be agreed. When, at the hospice where I work, the local Catholic curate was obviously uncomfortable with dying people and the whole concept of co-operation, and refused to make time even to meet the Medical Director, a Sister who worked in the parish became the eucharistic minister and pastoral visitor and in time was succeeded in that office by a long-term volunteer, who had taken early retirement from teaching. In the nature of things, clergy move on, and when a priest with training in hospice care was appointed as Catholic chaplain, the teamwork in the chaplaincy was restored. In as small a unit as a hospice, chaplains are noticed by other staff, and indeed they are quite closely and critically observed. If they simply pass each other by in the corridor, and never meet together, or confer about their ministry, this raises comment. If they come in, minister to one patient, and hurry out, this is seen as unacceptable behaviour. Chaplains are expected to meet and get to know the other staff, and this is good for them as well as for the morale of the unit.

CHURCH AND HOSPICE

There is another dimension to chaplaincy work and provision in many hospices, especially those who look to St Christopher's for inspiration. That the modern hospice movement had its origins in Christian concern for the welfare of the dying and that many of its founding mothers and fathers have been devoted members of their churches has been both a blessing and a disadvantage for chaplains. One would expect that the movement should be very chaplain-friendly, and it usually has been, but there have been times when it seemed that such ministry had to conform to the wishes of the founders and directors. In her biography of Cicely Saunders, Shirley du Boulay tellingly remarks: 'Cicely's relationship with the chaplain has never been an easy one. The chapel is the one place where she has no professional role . . . to be Chaplain at St Christopher's is no sinecure.'[2] Lay leaders of the movement have been inclined at times to equate Christianity with their own interpretation of it or with their particular church tradition. Conflicts have arisen with chaplains who have developed a more sophisticated and ecumenical outlook than that of their mentors to whom they would expect to look for encouragement and understanding. In a hospice with 'Christian' in its title, there might be a chaplain who feels he must challenge the model set up by the Trustees. Clergy, by reason of their training and experience, should have encountered a wide variety of expressions of the Christian faith, and should be open at least to trying to understand traditions which are quite alien to them. To enter chaplaincy and to be unable to recognize the faith of one's colleagues, let alone that of the rest of the staff and the patients, is to enter very dangerous territory.

SECULARIZATION AND SPIRITUALITY

We have already discussed in Chapter One something of the secularization process and its inevitable effect on the hospice movement. Here I want to concentrate on its 'churchly' attributes. Chaplaincy which sees itself as solely concerned with 'religion,' with sacraments and prayer and with talk about the faith, however valuable to some individuals, is not engaging with the reality of many patients' needs. Spirituality has become a very important concept in defining care. Physical, emotional and social care, along with spiritual care, are sometimes referred to as the four pillars of good hospice work.

But the 'spiritual' is very hard to define in this context. Sulmasy, in *The Healer's Calling*, defines spirituality as a description of 'one's relationship with God'.[3] But he acknowledges that this is not a universally acceptable definition. He is a doctor who is also a Franciscan Brother, so his definition is not unexpected, and it is refreshing since he is willing to be open about his faith. But it must be remembered that the spiritual is not the same as the religious, although it can and often is in practice still defined in terms of church membership and formal belief. If someone has a spiritual crisis, then 'send for the Chaplain', who is the expert. The official Circular *Meeting the Spiritual Needs of Patients and Staff*, designed to fulfil the Patients Charter in this area, suggests that the patient will be adequately provided for if she has access to a relevant minister of religion, of whatever creed. Provider units should decide how to meet the spiritual needs of patients and staff, by employing suitably qualified staff, contracting with relevant religious or spiritual organizations to provide equivalent services on a sessional or other basis, and facilitating access to patients by their religious leaders etc. Patients and staff should have reasonable facilities for religious observance such as a chapel or a prayer room, and the provision of whatever is necessary for worship. This suggests that nurses and others with intimate contact with patients are not primarily there to give spiritual care, and that should be left to the clergy. As Walter remarks, 'The activist nursing ethic of "getting through the work" contrasts strongly with ministry to the dying as espoused by many clergy, namely that it is a matter of "being with" or "being there" rather than of doing. Spiritual pain cannot be removed with a pill or with careful nursing . . . meeting spiritual needs by doing something – like calling the chaplain – fits the nursing ethos.'[4]

Definitions of 'spiritual' and of 'spirituality' are many and quite diverse. Spirituality could refer to the cultivation of the inner prayer life of the Christian and this is how it is still often used. It is an in-church concept. Even more in-church is the definition found in Canon Law of spirituality over against secular in terms of church property and administration. In nursing literature and increasingly in all healthcare discourse 'spirituality' is used as an alternative to 'religion', sometimes with the implication that religion is dated, constricting, frightening and generally not a good thing in the therapeutic process, whereas spirituality is open, wide-ranging, person-friendly and non-threatening, and belongs to everyone, patient and carer alike. We can all be spiritual. Now this may sound like a caricature, but it is how more traditional chaplains see the matter. I had thought that the word and concept of spirituality belonged to the philosophically literate chattering classes, until a new patient, speaking in a broad Edinburgh accent, remarked that he was not religious but 'awfie spiritual'. The concept has spread. But how do we define it? In the symposium *The Spiritual Challenge of Healthcare*, edited by Cobb and Robshaw, there are several attempts at a definition of spirituality. One is what they call a 'sparse' view of spirituality, which suggests that 'because being human is more than physical existence, and suffering is more than biological malfunction . . . there is what many people recognise as a spiritual quality to life which, in suffering, confronts people with questions and possibilities which reach beyond the immediate dilemmas of physical insult.'[5] In a later chapter Pamela Reed reports on research which allowed patients, nursing staff and chaplains to identify definitions of spirituality. 'Six categories were generated across all three groups. Two of these relate to the spirit component of transcendence: religious beliefs and activities, and contact with God. One category, values, related to both spirit and soul, with values such as health, freedom from guilt, hope, faith and the sacraments. The remaining three categories related to soul: relationships with others, affective experiences like peace and comfort); and communication abilities.'[6] This survey interestingly intermingles spiritual and religious, and introduces yet another concept, that of the soul. In another chapter on spirituality and world faiths, Ian Markham reminds us how easy it is to be limited to Christian and post-Christian societies when describing spirituality. Having borrowed Linda Ross's description of spirituality as 'the need for: meaning, purpose and fulfilment in life; hope/will to live; belief and faith', he goes on to point out that not all faith systems recognize the concept, and that much translation is often necessary.[7]

At the very least it has to be admitted that we are dealing with slippery definitions here. We all, in our different professions, know what we mean by spirituality, but definition is almost impossible.

In these conditions, and with this expressed scepticism, can the hospice help in defining spirituality, and in delivering spiritual care to the dying and their families? Because it is a small and intimate unit, where doctors and nurses have more time to spend holding patients' hands and listening to their real anxieties, and because there are often chaplains who are able and willing to share their insights with other staff and to respect their observations, I believe that there is a contribution the movement can make. But before I discuss this it is necessary to arrive at a few definitions. We have seen that there is a common if misguided understanding that spiritual needs can be met by religious means. The opposing tendency is to reject talk of religious needs because of the connotations of church with all its imperfections, and what to many carers seems its irrelevance in the present time. It is helpful for clarity to draw up lists of religious and spiritual needs. This at least gives a basis for discussion.

Spiritual needs
- Being valued
- Finding meaning in life and death
- Being aware of love and care

- Being listened to
- Being treated as more than a sick body

Religious needs
- Prayer
- Bible reading
- Religious person, e.g. clergyman
- Sacraments
- Holy objects, e.g. crucifix, rosary
- Religious books and pamphlets
- Access to a specifically religious place, e.g. chapel with Christian symbols and/or the symbols of another faith
- The possibility of discussing funeral services and spirituality

Walter quotes Cicely Saunders: 'We can always persevere with the practical. Care for the physical needs; the time taken to elucidate a symptom, the quiet acceptance of a family's angry demands, the way nursing care is given, can carry it all and reach the most hidden places. This may be all we can offer to "inarticulate" spiritual pain – it may well be enough as our patients finally face the truth on the other side of death.'
He comments that this definition of spiritual care

is wide enough to allow chaplains and nurses to squabble over rights to its practice. Nurses who emphasise that spiritual care is part of the nurse's task of caring for the whole patient define it in this broad way and try to restrict chaplains and clergy to more formal religious activities, such as taking church services and praying with patients. Chaplains however don't usually find it satisfying to restrict their role to that of ritual specialists, claiming instead to be experts in helping patients seek meaning.[8]

PASTORAL CARE

So where do spirituality and pastoral care, which is presumably what the chaplain believes he can offer, coincide? Pastoral care has been defined in several ways. It is based on individuals, it is active and comprehensive. This means that it is personal, trust creating, listening, and possibly non-judgemental. It is also rooted in faith, whether that is made explicit or not, and it is willing to make use of the Christian story in its encounter with spiritual distress.[9] The presence of a chaplain implies that the hospice wishes to give patients and families access to the resources of the Christian faith, and while she is aware of the nature of spirituality, and the longings of people who cannot articulate their faith, the chaplain is always conscious of a specific commitment to her faith community. This statement might well be contested by some, who would see the chaplain's task as to meet people where they are and not in any way to intrude her own beliefs and doubts. Yet this attitude seems to negate the need for specifically 'religious' persons being involved in the care of the dying. Certainly the frontiers of the institutional church are shrinking, and younger patients are less likely to have a living connection with the church, but that in itself does not absolve chaplains from their commitment to the faith. Pastoral care is not evangelism, nor is the chaplain called to be an evangelist, but she is a witness to what we may dare to call a transcendent world.

WORSHIP IN THE HOSPICE

The most obvious exercise of a chaplain's gifts is in the conduct of formal worship, and the giving of the sacraments. Services can be held in the chapel, if one is available, at the bedside, in the quiet room, or wherever opportunity arises. In St Christopher's prayers have been broadcast to the wards, and patients may listen or not. In St Columba's in Edinburgh, in the early days, some nurses trained in English hospitals where ward prayers were still said volunteered to read a short prayer in the rooms each morning. When the governing body heard of this, it decreed its immediate cessation. 'There will be no compulsory prayers here!' And indeed Scots were embarrassed. They do their religion at home and in private, and are not always comfortable with too much publicity. The whole incident made us think carefully about the messages conveyed by the presence of a chapel and a chaplaincy team, and we have tried not to allow distinctions to arise between those patients in the Day Hospice who choose to attend morning prayers in the chapel and those who prefer not to do so.

A designated worship area certainly makes matters easier. It can be used as a quiet retreat, or a place for intimate family conversation. It can also be used for public worship. Services are short, bearing in mind that attention span is limited in very ill people. They are attended by patients, visitors, volunteers and staff, and, in the hospice which I know well, are, on Sundays, services of Holy Communion. The presupposition is that touch and taste, and familiar words and gestures will convey far more to dying people than a formal sermon. This may hardly need to be said in many places, but the Scottish Presbyterian tradition of very infrequent communion, perhaps two or four times annually in many parishes, raises the occasional query from patients. 'But I came to communion last week!' To offset this startled outburst of surprise, many have commented gratefully on the opportunity to share the service as a family, or perhaps to take part for the first time in their lives, and many patients have for long been too ill and uncomfortable to attend their own churches.

This raises the question of church discipline. I have already stressed the importance of being closely linked with the wider church. So dare unconfirmed persons take communion? What does the Protestant chaplain do if a Catholic patient holds out his hand when she approaches with the bread and wine? A hospice chapel is not the place to make ecumenical experiments, but it is emphatically not the place to turn anyone away from the gifts of God. Antonio was a flamboyant Italian patient, who noticed the chaplain celebrating communion at the bedside of a woman who belonged to the Christian Brethren. Her son, a member of the Church of Scotland, was there, and this was significant, as he said afterwards that he had not been permitted to break bread with his mother since he had left the Brethren as a young man. Antonio approached and asked to be included in the service. A Religious Sister, who was a flower volunteer that afternoon, looked a little alarmed, and said to him, 'Don't you see it's a Protestant service?' 'If I am offered Christ, how can I refuse?'

replied Antonio. Now in this incident several ecclesiastical
legalities may have been infringed, but it is surely in the spirit
of hospice care to act immediately, and not to ask questions,
and I trust it is in the spirit of the Jesus of the Gospels, who
was notorious for mixing in all sorts of company, and bringing
God's presence and forgiveness to all sorts of people. Here
hospice care, faith and ecclesiastical practice converge in a
very acute manner. There is no time to make references to
textbooks of Canon Law or even to living authorities. When a
fellow-human asks for bread and wine the chaplain may not
refuse, not be seen to hesitate or be judgemental. The time for
reflection is later. Desert-island theology, doing what must be
done, following the spontaneity of Jesus is called for. This is not
to say that emergency situations ought to become routine, nor
that we should extrapolate from one incident a new policy
of intercommunion, but *in extremis* (and the hospice is a
place of extreme and unforeseen situations) we must be able
to react with believing flexibility.

How obviously Christian may a hospice chapel be? There
are those who would fear offence if there were any Christian
symbols or even the use of the word 'chapel'. Certainly there
should be no intention of excluding members of other faith
communities from all aspects of hospice care, and conditions
are very different in various parts of the British Isles. But there
is a danger in attempting to be so all-inclusive that something
vital to the majority of our patients is lost. The very name
'chapel' has in the west of Scotland certain strong connotations. It is a word only applied to Roman Catholic places of
worship. This is not so much so in the east of Scotland, and in
England and Wales 'chapel' is usually a Nonconformist church
building, but I have met folk who were astonished to find
themselves, as they thought, at Catholic worship, because it
took place in the 'chapel'.

At the other Christian extreme, it was suggested that many
Catholic patients would not be happy in the chapel unless the
reserved sacrament was present, with a sanctuary light as a
focus. The first Catholic chaplain held this view, and as soon
as it was expressed and discussed in the Chaplaincy Advisory
Committee the Bishop of Edinburgh in the Scottish Episcopal

Church said, 'If they have it, so must we!' We were faced with the prospect of rival tabernacles, and the predominantly Presbyterian Board of Governors dismissed the idea, as did the next Catholic chaplain, and the matter has never been raised again. In the vestry of our fairly new custom-built chapel are two lockable wooden wall cupboards, labelled Episcopalian and Roman Catholic, which could serve as aumbries, and so far as I am aware they have never been so used.

Christians from many denominations have attended worship together both at morning prayers, and on Sundays for communion, and have felt themselves bound together by the fact that they are in the one caring unit. Some who I know would keep very carefully to their own ways of worship outside have had no difficulty with a shared service in the chapel. Catholic patients are offered communion daily at their bedside or on the veranda, and other patients sitting nearby have been heard to join in the 'Our Father'. For a few years on Maundy Thursday we attempted a joint Eucharist, or rather three running concurrently, as a student attached to the chaplaincy irreverently described the event. The (Protestant) chaplain celebrated communion, and the Catholic and Episcopalian priests served their people with consecrated bread. It seemed a good idea to demonstrate on that of all days that we were servants of one Jesus, and a number of staff and volunteers who were working at the time of the services in their own churches would attend. But several of them objected to the seating arrangements: Catholics on the right, Episcopalians on the left, and all the rest in the middle. They deliberately sat in the wrong place! Soon after this happened we decided to drop the practice.

Ministers and priests are encouraged to use the chapel for family services, and adherents of quite exclusive bodies, such as the True Jesus Chinese Church, and the Church of Jesus Christ of the Latter-Day Saints, have found no difficulty in using the chapel as a meeting space.

Occasionally Jewish patients have attended prayers, presumably to see how we do it, and there is an embroidery of our logo, complete with cross and dove, on one of our walls which is the gift and handiwork of an Orthodox Jew whose father and mother-in-law died in our care. It may be that we become over-anxious lest we offend members of other faith-communities, to the extent that we hide our true faith. Chaplains are not indeed appointed to evangelize, but we cannot pretend to be what we are not or not to be what we are. We are not social workers with clerical collars, but servants of Christ in a particular and complex calling.

PASTORAL CARE

'How do you approach a patient?'

'Do you only go if you are called, or do you speak to everyone?'

'Do you ever get turned away?'

'Do many dying people turn to God and repent?'

Questions like these come fairly constantly from students of various disciplines, from friends and colleagues, and from the occasional researcher who is writing a book on hospice care. Some codes of practice promise a visit from the chaplain within 24 or 48 hours. Other hospices are more relaxed about this. For some people it would be quite alarming to be confronted by the chaplain within a few hours of arriving in this strange new place, but for most folk today the image of the chaplain as the one who precedes the undertaker down the ward is no longer a real one. They are so unaccustomed to seeing a minister that they may be quite curious to explore a new relationship. Of course there are patients who ask to meet the chaplain as a priority, and others who on no account wish to see such a person, but they are few. Generally, in such a small place, it is possible to know when new patients have arrived and indeed to have some information about them. If it seems appropriate, an early contact is made, and in the course of a few days all patients will have been at least spoken to briefly.

Sometimes relatives ask that no chaplain go near the patient, usually because there is some fear about what the patient can bear to know about her illness, and such patients often do welcome a meeting in due time. It is remarkable how little relatives know about the family religious experience. Every time I approached an old man whose wife was in constant attendance, he would begin to explain why he never went to church. 'I believe in God all right. You can worship God anywhere. You don't need a special building,' he would say, as a sort of automatic response to my presence; and his wife would say, 'Jimmy, we've been married 40 years and you've never talked to me about that.'

If a patient refuses to see a chaplain, then his wishes must be observed. I think that has happened to me no more than three or four times in more than 20 years. A chaplain is a non-threatening presence to most folk. She will not produce a needle, or prescribe a pill. She will go away when she is told to go, and there are various techniques for giving this message, such as continuing to read the newspaper, keeping on the headphones, or in one case, producing the mobile phone and explaining that a business call was on its way from Greece. She will also sit for as long as needed, and listen, and pray or do whatever is required at the time, which may be to pour a drink of water, or discuss the Test Match, or listen to complaints about the other patients, or the staff!

A chaplain needs a good supply of apparently trivial talk. This can be a hard lesson to learn. We feel so privileged to be close to dying folk, that it may seem wrong to talk about the flowers, the family or the football match or indeed about oneself in answer to questions, but these topics are the small change of human relationships, and convey shared humanity. What appear to be trivia are possibly the only vocabulary that can be used to communicate. It is not so much the words but the manner of the chaplain that may win confidence. After apparent trivia, in which the chaplain is quietly being assessed, come the real questions, the agonies and tears, the smiles and reassurances. In my first days as a hospice chaplain I attended a prayer meeting, and listened to a devout fellow-Baptist pray that I would snatch many brands from the burning. This image, of the guardian at the gates of hell, continues to haunt my less than conscious self, however much I repudiate such theology. But I know that I am not called to be an evangelist in that sense, and I have rediscovered the strength of the Calvinist doctrine of the sovereignty of God.

So, do many turn to God? In my experience few in so many words. There are those who go back to their Sunday School lessons or to the days at the Boys' Brigade Bible Class, and who rebuild a childhood faith which has been overlaid by the cares and pleasures of this world. There are others who ask the chaplain what she believes, about God, and about life after death, and of course there are many who can talk quite easily about our shared faith and hopes and fears. But actual death-bed conversions are not common. It may be that by the time patients get to a hospice all such matters have been settled. It may be that many patients are having so much trouble to concentrate and to breathe and say a few words, that much is left unsaid.

Colin had been in the Boys' Brigade attached to the chaplain's church, many years before. He had lapsed from any form of religious activity when he got married, and he was pleased when old men from the church who remembered him as a boy came to visit. He said little to the chaplain, until one Sunday he appeared at the service, and took communion. 'I'll tell you about it tomorrow,' he said, but the next day he became unconscious holding the hands of his 'two Marys,' one his common-law wife, and the other the very distinguished minister of the church to which his wife had been nominally attached. The next day he died.

Colin's story illustrates one of the most difficult and frustrating parts of hospice chaplaincy. We never hear the end of the story. One day we are talking, we have to go, and the next day it is too late, and the illness has progressed. Hints are dropped, coded language used, but the chaplain has to learn to leave outcomes in the hands of God. Dame Cicely has many stories of dying people who have changed in their attitude to God in their last days, and any chaplain could tell the same, but for every open conversation, there must be hundreds that are inconclusive, tangential, apparently without much depth. Then you will be told by the relatives, 'She did enjoy her little chats with you.' And you wonder what has been going on.

Sometimes it is just native reticence that stops spiritual conversation. A student for the priesthood of the Church of England on a longer course was assigned to a reasonably fit patient who was known to be a regular church attender. All Peter would tell the young man was that going to church helped him, and then he would change the subject and talk about football. One day Peter's minister came to visit him, and said to the chaplain on the way out, 'There's a great Christian!'

'Tell that to my student.'

'But', said the minister, 'he's a Scot! We don't wear our religion on our sleeve.'

Whether this is really a national characteristic or a convenient myth I am not sure, since I was brought up in evangelical circles, where we were encouraged to be almost embarrassingly open about the need for conversion and the joys of the Christian life. But those of us who were encouraged to talk about our faith openly and aggressively find reticence, and vague sounding beliefs, and indifference, difficult to accept, and have to curb our desire to evangelize.

IMPLICIT AND EXPLICIT RELIGION

As we have seen, definitions of religion and spirituality are elusive. Many who would describe themselves as not religious would claim to be spiritual, and some observers would contend that everyone is a spiritual being and will in some way respond to the right approach. The concept of implicit religion is of help in shedding light on this question. As described by Edward Bailey, to whose Network for the Study of Implicit Religion I owe a great deal, the concept of implicit religion counterbalances the tendency to equate 'religion' with specialized institutions, with articulated beliefs, and with that which is consciously willed (or specifically intended).[10] This approach, according to Bailey,

> opens up the possibility of discovering the sacred within what otherwise might be dismissed as profane, and of finding an experience of the holy within an apparently irreligious realm. Above all, in contemporary society it allows for the discovery of some kind of religiosity within what conventionally might be seen as an unrelievedly secular sphere. The concept therefore gives credence to the

opinion of the 'person in the street' – 'that while some who go to church really mean it, others who go to church really have a different religion altogether' – but that everybody has a religion of some sort, a faith by which they live, albeit as an unconscious core at the centre of their way of life and being.[11]

This recognition of core values as being of ultimate importance is of great help in hospice ministry. Certainly many who profess Christianity and go to church regularly have beliefs that complement or contradict the official teachings of their churches. It seems to be quite possible to sing the hymns about the resurrection and secretly believe in reincarnation, to say the Apostles' Creed and to have grave doubts about the virgin birth or life after death. Private faith sometimes surfaces when people are very ill, and they become aware of discrepancies, but also of what they hold most dear.

'I believe in the hospice way of life,' may seem a strange credo, yet there are those who have found an implicit religion in the philosophy of living until you die. More likely implicit beliefs in family values, in friendship, or in the innate goodness of the universe will comfort and sustain people. People must be encountered where they are, and not where we would like them to be, and facing death makes for an appraisal of what is really significant. Communities other than church are supportive. It is noticeable how many uniformed members of the bowling club turn up at the funeral of a member. Chrissie and her husband had been keen cyclists, going off with the cycling club every weekend, and so lapsing from church. When I asked if their two sons were also cyclists I was told that they had been 'brought up in the faith', and at Chrissie's funeral were a significant number of women and men in cycling gear. For her and her family cycling was not a substitute for religion. It could be described, without any sense of irony, as 'the faith'. It was a form of implicit religion, and as such gave meaning to their lives.

It is quite fascinating to disentangle what people really believe from what they think they ought to say when the minister visits. This certainly poses a problem for the Christian pastor, whose instinct may be to correct and try to change what she sees as error. Just as life is being stripped down by the approach of death, and movement and initiative are being gradually restricted, so the trimmings of outward religion may fade, the exclusiveness and sometimes the assurance that one is right become eroded, and core beliefs, which really matter and give meaning, emerge.

A COMMUNITY OF CARE

The Anabaptist/Mennonite model of the church, as a community of committed people, covenanted together in baptism to be the people of God, and resisting hierarchical models of organization, has been seen as a useful model in congregational life in many publications in the last few years. This represents a rediscovery of one of the oldest strands of Christian community life, with its roots in the Radical Reformation. To be church is to be mutually caring. Richard Hays, while not explicitly Anabaptist, in his book *The Moral Vision of the New Testament*, shows how this might be possible in the particular case of a church family faced with a question of an abortion. He writes:

> the church should follow the example of the compassionate Samaritan, of the early Jerusalem church and of Jesus himself, all of whom acted sacrificially for the sake of others, particularly those who were weak, poor or helpless. To act in imaginative response to these paradigms would bring the church into new practices of community and new relations to neighbours not previously acknowledged as neighbours.[12]

I would contend that the hospice is most churchlike when it acts as a community of professional and volunteer, carer and cared-for, as an institution which attends to those who are unlikeable, isolated and condemned by society. This must sound very idealistic, for many of those concerned are not acting directly from Christian motives, and many patients would not appreciate being considered unlikeable and condemned. Yet a compassionate reaction, in medical care, in nursing, in the pouring of a cup of water, in holding a hand, is surely a response, implicitly or explicitly, to the demands of the Christian gospel. The hospice movement, sometimes very openly, sometimes covertly, is a consciously Christian one, however secularization may have swept in, and so long as there continues to be a community response to the needs of the weak, it will continue to witness to the virtues of non-hierarchical co-operation in care.

It should also be evident that care is shown in many different dimensions. Patients watch one another, and can quite movingly become involved in the illness of a neighbour, whether they feel able to talk and listen to the other, or whether they only know when to call for nursing help. Visitors come to know each other, and often attend funerals of their new friends, and continue to keep in touch with the family. At quarterly services of remembrance, whole groups of relatives sometimes meet and exchange experiences. Thus patients and relatives themselves form a caring community. Similarly in the Day Hospice, the 'Monday' folk can sometimes become closely bonded. When one of them enters the nursing wing, they will make the short journey to visit, and when one dies, they will mourn as a group.

There can grow up a strong sense of solidarity among the staff, and among volunteers, and one of the chaplain's duties and delights is to be a pastor to those she works with. This may involve hearing troubled consciences, or conducting the wedding of a nurse, or the funeral of the relative of a volunteer. When the chaplain herself is in need or bereaved, the hospice community can be a great strength. All these actions reflect the activities of a living church, and can indeed provide a paradigm for congregational life.

THE QUESTIONS OF THE DYING

'Do people have specific questions?' I am asked by visiting students. It would be convenient to produce a list, with appropriate answers! And there are areas where questions occur with some regularity. 'Why me?' is the most obvious. The unfairness of life, and the apparently random nature of cancer evoke this response, sometimes in the context of asking why the man next door, who does all the things I have abstained from, seems to be healthy. It would be possible to attempt philosophical answers, to discourse on the life and death patterns evident in the universe, to speak of being made from the dust of destroyed stars, and of being recycled as part of God's great plan for creation. I suspect such discourse would not be very productive. Indeed I have come to believe that the asking of the question is enough. The chaplain is not expected to have the answer. Sometimes a patient will talk about this and say that he has been able to say, 'Why not me?' But to reach that stage of acceptance is a gift not given to many. It is not only the patients who ask this question and it is the task of the chaplain to listen to the family, and to agree that there is apparent unfairness and certainly a great mystery here.

'Will God accept me?' is an interestingly open question, and it may conceal a sense of guilt and unworthiness that has its beginnings in childhood experiences, or in a particular theology. So long as life seems to go on without too many incidents this question can be put aside, but the imminence of death forces confrontation with the possibility of rejection. The response depends on what the chaplain knows of the person. Reassurance of God's unlimited love, stories of Jesus, and prayers, may be the most effective answers. For other people there is required an exploration of the past, and possibly the bringing to light of events long almost forgotten. Men who have been in the wars of the last century still carry heavy burdens and unquiet thoughts that can return in nightmares when death approaches.

Sometimes questions appear as challenges. 'I've never done Him any harm, why should He harm me?' is a not untypical way of testing out the chaplain. The innate Pelagianism of the Briton is often evident. 'I've done my best, and I've not harmed anyone.' And who can deny this, on a short acquaintance? Yet Christianity offers forgiveness on the basis of what God has done for us in Christ. So a chaplain has to build on the positive, and gently suggest that perhaps life has not been quite perfect.

It is a commonplace of hospice experience that patients do not fear death, but rather the dying process. The dread of losing control over the mind, and over bodily functions, the spectre of unbearable pain or of choking to death are far more real than a fear of judgement or of the afterlife. Only very occasionally has anyone asked me about hell, and heaven often seems to be defined as the very best hour spent with the most beloved person, prolonged infinitely. Yet I am convinced that behind many other questions there lurks a fear of punishment, darkness or annihilation. As secularization advances there has indeed been an 'eclipse of eternity,' and our ancestors would be surprised at the insouciance with which we contemplate the beyond, but belief in an afterlife is by no means extinct, as Tony Walter and others have shown.[13]

One reaction to the realization that death is imminent is to seek to be reconciled with the church. Many a lapsed Catholic has gratefully received the sacraments and returned to the faith. Occasionally I have been asked to baptize a patient, and several grandchildren have been christened 'before granny dies'. Patients seek to have a civil marriage blessed, or indeed a long-term relationship regularized, in the hospice chapel. I have already mentioned the power of the offer of bread and wine. Who knows what spiritual journeys the dying accomplish, surprising their friends and discovering for themselves a rebirth of faith?

FOR FURTHER THOUGHT

1 Is it harmful to think of the hospice as a substitute church? Does this not have value in a changing society?

2 Need a hospice chaplain have a live connection with a local church? Is this a matter of theology or of personal taste?

NOTES

1 Shirley du Boulay, *Cicely Saunders*. London: Hodder & Stoughton 1984, p. 162.
2 *Ibid.*
3 D. P. Sulmasy, *The Healer's Calling*. New York/Makoyah New Jersey: Paulist Press 1997, p. 10.
4 Tony Walter, *The Revival of Death*. London: Routledge 1994, p. 100.

5 Mark Cobb and Vanessa Robshaw, eds., *The Spiritual Challenge of Health Care*. Edinburgh: Churchill Livingstone 1998, pp. 1-2.

6 *Op. cit.*, p. 43.

7 *Op. cit.*, p. 74.

8 *Op. cit.*, p. 102.

9 For further discussion, see Alastair V. Campbell, *Rediscovering Pastoral Care* (2nd edn, Darton Longman & Todd 1986), and David Lyall, *Integrity of Pastoral Care* (SPCK 2001).

10 In William H. Swatos, ed., *Encyclopedia of Religion and Society*. Lanham, Maryland: AltaMira 1998, p. 235. Cf. also Edward I. Bailey, *Implicit Religion in Contemporary Society*. Kampen, Netherlands: Kok Pharos 1997. Also Wesley Carr, *Handbook of Pastoral Studies*. London: SPCK 1997, pp. 208-9.

11 William H. Swatos, ed., *op. cit.*, p. 236.

12 Richard B. Hays, *The Moral Vision of the New Testament*. Edinburgh: T. & T. Clark 1997, p. 456.

13 Tony Walter, *The Eclipse of Eternity: a Sociology of the Afterlife*. Basingstoke: Macmillan 1996.

CHAPTER FOUR

The Hospice as Home

In this chapter I want to look at the hospice unit as I have experienced it for over twenty years, as firstly a part-time member of staff, then for fourteen years wholetime chaplain, and also as a person who has had a number of relatives and friends among the patients. I was born and brought up in Edinburgh, and returned to a small city centre church in 1973. In 1977 I was appointed as part-time chaplain to the new experiment, St Columba's Hospice, which, although it was predated by Marie Curie Homes, and the NHS Roxburgh Houses in Aberdeen and Dundee, was the first independent unit in the St Christopher's tradition. With impressive arrogance some founding members of staff gave a series of lectures on hospice care to other newly appointed staff and to volunteers, some of whom had been working hard at fund- and consciousness-raising for several years. Then we held a service in the local parish church, and with trepidation awaited the first patient. This would prove that there was need for a hospice, that GPs might actually make use of it, and that our building, a Georgian house on the edge of the Firth of Forth, would be capable of caring for patients.

The first patient was Jack, a retired sailor whose daughter had become weary with caring for him. He looked out over the water from his bed, and enjoyed the attentions of nurses and volunteers, and the skill of the doctor. His daughter came to visit, they talked late into the night and they were apparently reconciled, and then he died peacefully. It was a textbook case. Friendly and familiar surroundings evoking nostalgic conversations, problems with relationships overcome, time to

talk, quiet death: they were all there. I would like to say that
he made his peace with God with the help of the devoted
chaplain, possibly at 3 a.m., but I cannot find that in my
memory! Of course in the first weeks we entertained as our
patients complaining folk, unconscious folk, grand and patronizing ladies and all the rest. At least our early experience
reminded us of the principles of our foundation, that we
should care for people with 'terminal' illness in as homelike
an atmosphere as possible.

'Hospice' is derived from the Latin word *hospitium*, which
has the meaning both of host and of guest. The hospice is
designed to be a place of hospitality, practised in mutuality.
Just as in our own homes there can be a welcoming atmosphere and careful preparation, and it can all be wasted on
ungrateful, unhappy or insensitive guests, so in a hospice
there needs to be both the welcome and a willing acceptance
of the need for care. This is a difficult ideal to realize. Some
guests are hard to like, and many arrive against their will,
under pressure from carers or consultants, and sometimes
they are not aware of the nature of the institution, or have a
false idea of it. Yet the sharing of hospitality happens, as
patients settle to the regime of treatment, rest and stimula-
tion. When visitors arrive they can be greeted by staff of all
sorts, informed about the patient and the institution, and
made to feel useful.

In early days it was laid down that one of the criteria for
entry was lack of any community support. In any city there
are lodging houses, where for one reason or another people
have found refuge. To be discharged from hospital with
advanced cancer into a bare room, which in some cases has to
be vacated during the day, is a bleak prospect. The excellent
medical service which cares for these institutions occasionally
refers people to our place of hospitality. Joe was well educated.
Indeed his old school tie, which both the Medical Director
and the chaplain also had the right to wear, was always neatly
rolled on his locker, and seemed his link with respectability.
He had been a research scientist, and had gradually become
estranged from his family, so that when he arrived he claimed
that he had no next-of-kin. For some years he had spent

Wednesday nights in the hall of the church where I had been minister. There with others he had found friendship, dominoes and sandwiches, and from time to time he had disappeared for long periods. 'Joe's on a bender,' I would hear from Kate who ran the evening. Then one day he appeared at St Columba's, dignified, ill and quiet. Volunteers arrived with a cup of tea, nurses took details, doctors did tests, the chaplain looked surprised and I hope welcoming. And Joe said nothing. He disappeared for long periods, which is not very easy in such a busy place. He would be found locked in the visitors' shower room, or wandering in the grounds, or anywhere he could be alone. To extend hospitality to such a solitary man was a challenge. Gradually he became weaker, and spent more time in bed. Nurses won his confidence. We discovered his sister living not far away, and some sort of family reunion took place.

Joe is only one of our city's wanderers whom we have cared for. Perhaps he is an extreme case, but he is typical of those who have felt rejected by family and old friends, who have been ashamed of their lifestyle, and who have been to some extent addicted to alcohol or drugs. Hospices are accused of having a middle-class ambience, and of being very respectable and even holy places. The dangers of being patronizing and judgemental are always there. Certainly we like our patients to be well washed, and afternoon tea is served in china cups. Yet the potential for acceptance, for sympathetic listening, can bring even a shy and enclosed man like Joe back to some peace. Joe also reminds us how much there is that is secret in every life, and how that secrecy may be relaxed in the presence of death.

Hospitality has no bounds of human class and temperament. It extends to the 'difficult' patient and her family, to the ungrateful, and to the uncomprehending. It requires effort by staff and volunteers, and it can be remarkably rewarding. To see a frightened and hostile patient relax and begin to feel comfortable, even for brief periods, is very satisfying. Giving and receiving hospitality is one of the ways in which the hospice, even if unconsciously, mirrors the gospel. The early church practised hospitality for travelling preachers and all who arrived in the name of Christ.[1] The church set out to be a community rooted in the unconditional love of God. Homes and meals, talking and listening, support in times of trouble are marks of a living community, and to be true to its origins, the hospice must provide more than a medical and nursing service. It must practise *hospitium*.

Jennifer Hockey, in her anthropologically based account *Experiences of Death*, gives a vivid description of the arrival of a new day patient at Strathcarron Hospice, in the Central Region of Scotland.

> A larger crowd than usual gathers on a Friday morning in the sombre wood-panelled room at the end of Strathcarron's central corridor. Voluntary chauffeurs, homely, middle-class women and a few retired men, have brought them from home to the foot of the outside steps. A wheelchair or a supporting arm steers them into the pine-scented hallway, wood panelled too and dimly lit. . . . Among these passengers many have cancer and most are expected to die within months. . . . Prints of waves breaking, of Impressionist yachts at sunset, ease the passage into a hallway/stairwell reception area. Here a mosaic impression of handcraft and medicine confronts the patient. The carefully sustained, seemingly limitless warmth of their voluntary chauffeur is now mirrored in the greeting of a voluntary receptionist. Embroidering or knitting patch blankets, the receptionist is framed within a scene of 'Guess-my-Birthday' baby dolls; a glimpsed sluice room; inert, crochet-blanketed bodies; and collapsed, waiting wheelchairs. Rarely empty, this space is a meeting point. Four doorways and the staircase provide entry for sombre-suited doctors, administrators, undertakers and the Chaplain; for white and blue uni-formed female nurses and domestics; and for less readily identifiable female home-care nurses, voluntary helpers and the social worker. Loudly humorous greetings and a quieter and more urgent exchange of messages merge in an atmosphere of heady seriousness. Threading their way through this public space towards toilets and lounge, in-patients may sometimes be identified by dressing gown or

by hand-held catheter bag. In other cases slippers and slow tread are the only indications.

Hockey goes on to describe a day in the hospice. It finishes with an outdoor singsong, which she describes as hovering 'delicately between the wildly farcical and the desperately tragic'.[2]

This account, while perhaps a little too dramatic, nevertheless touches on several aspects of the hospice as home. There is the mixture of staff, volunteers and patients in a small space where little can be hidden, the humorous and occasionally anxious attempt to make the best of things, and the unavoidable intrusion of the medical apparatus into normal conversation and activities.

Katherine Froggatt, in an article in the journal *Mortality*,[3] writes of the hospice as standing on the *limen* between life and death. The state of liminality lies in a strange and dangerous place between the known and the unknown. Those who occupy this space are ritually unclean and symbolically dangerous to those outside the *limen*.[4] She points out that access to hospice care involves crossing a boundary which marks the entry to liminal space, from the secular to the sacred, and once admitted the patient effectively enters into the experience of *communitas*, where relationships no longer are based on hierarchy but on equality. Hospice care speaks of a journey, and the crossing of a threshold. Not only is the dying person and her family welcomed and cared for, but she is encouraged on her life journey, and the family are incorporated in the bereavement follow-up and after-care. Liminality implies absence of status, and the patient and her kin are encouraged to see the hospice as 'family'. Froggatt quotes from the literature of an unnamed hospice in Hampshire:

A Hospice environment resembles a family, with the patient regarded as the much loved member of the family who has come to stay with his/her adoptive parents, the hospice team providing the extended family figures. Family life, as we are all aware, is not all harmony; periods of discontent do occur. But with the commitment of the team to good internal and outside communication, the primary aim of St Elsewhere's Hospice to 'serve the needs of the dying and their families' will be achieved.[5]

Froggatt points out that the images of family in hospice literature are often fragmentary and selective. The hospice can scarcely promote the more negative aspects of family life, the anger and division all too common in our experience. Perhaps within the liminal space, the mysterious area between living and dying, it is necessary to overstress the positive aspects of family life.

In our own homes we dress as we please. That is one of the marks of home. In an effort to be homelike questions have been raised about uniforms in hospice circles. Doctors seem more at ease in their white coats, which keep their day clothes clean and provide pockets for the essential stethoscope, and nurses need to be distinguished by what they wear. Uniform, provided by the hospice, saves cleaning bills on ordinary clothes. After several votes over a few years, the nurses at St Columba's abandoned wearing hats, and nobody complained. All staff and volunteers wear badges, and one of the ways in which a hospice is not homelike is in its insistence on tight security. There are self-locking doors, alarms, digital entry devices and all the trappings of an institution, although many of the patients will have come from sheltered housing, with similar precautions, or from private homes with an alarm system. As drugs are stored in a hospice, and there are valuable computer systems, and as even such a place, loved by the whole community, is targeted by folk with intent to steal, great care is necessary.

On the other hand, one of the things that makes a house a home is privacy. We can shut the door, and even switch off the telephone, and we are safe. In a hospice privacy is possible. Intruders are kept out, visitors can be controlled in number and length of stay, there are private interview and rest rooms, and locks on the toilet doors. Yet inevitably in shared rooms conversations are overheard, and one patient can become very interested in the lives and troubles of the rest. Some patients and their families need single rooms, and those who stay for a longer period sometimes have quite a lot of their own possessions brought in. Others prefer the company of a shared room. It is not always easy for staff to guess which kind of room new patients will want. Occasionally a patient lays down the provision of a single room as a condition of coming in, for a variety of good and less good reasons. Quite often patients simply go where there is a bed, and make the best of things, and there are those who first choose to be on their own, and then become lonely and are glad to transfer to a bigger area. In her provocative book, *The Dying Process*, Julia Lawton suggests that single rooms are preferred by middle-class patients and that those from lower social groupings enjoy company more. This has certainly not been my experience.[6] The choices made are far more complex or sometimes for-tuitous. They may depend upon the bedstate on the day of admission, or on expressed preference. Division on class lines has not been evident, although certainly many professional people, doctors, nurses and clergy in particular, prefer privacy. But generalization is impossible.

'A SMALL PLACE'

In describing a hospice to those who have never visited one, I often hear myself saying 'a small place'. This might sound disparaging, as if small were unimportant. Certainly it is small compared with the great city hospitals, but in fact with 30 beds St Columba's is a large hospice. When the Day Hospice and the Education Unit are added, along with all the offices, it is quite a complex building. Yet it remains smallscale. There are no plans to have more beds and the building programme seems to be complete, at least for the moment. Perhaps a better word than 'small' is 'manageable'. It is possible to get lost in the buildings, but not for long. Although there are over 100 staff and up to 400 volunteers most folk know one another. There is, we like to claim, a 'family feeling'. This has persisted despite many changes, and especially the building of the nursing wing, which to some extent separated the nursing from the administrative staff, and was greeted with nostalgic sighs by those on the staff who wanted the place to remain really intimate. But even now there are no long corridors, the kitchens are relatively near the wards, and the appearance and indeed the reality of working as one unit are maintained. Because we are a relatively small place we are more able to practise hospitality. Adventurous patients, who are mobile enough, can explore the building, and are encouraged to do so, so that they feel they know it.

Most hospices are set in attractive grounds. In Edinburgh the Fairmile Marie Curie Centre is on the southern edge of the city, in the foothills of the Pentlands. St Columba's is on the northern shore, overlooking the Forth and the coastal towns of Fife. Gardens, with their variety of trees and flowers, are wonderful for walking in, and just observing. A previous owner of Challenger Lodge laid out its grounds with quite exotic trees and shrubs. Over the years and with varied occupation, this garden receded, but we are left with a large Cedar of Lebanon, which must be approaching 200 years old, and is a constant source of delight. Add to the garden the white doves, the squirrels, an occasional fox, and a large dog, and there is plenty to see and comment on.

A few years ago a rather informal nursery for the children of staff was rebuilt to meet government regulations, the volunteer helpers gave way to trained nursery nurses, and local children joined the children of staff and sometimes of patients. Endless entertainment is provided for patients watching children at play. Just occasionally it is assumed, usually by well-meaning visitors, that the children are also ill, but a few moments' observation disproves that theory!

Light colours, carefully chosen furniture, comfortable reclining chairs, and well-maintained property all add to the sense of welfare and care. This begins to sound like the script for a promotional video, but it is important to stress that such apparently trivial matters enhance the quality of care. From my own observation this could be said of all hospices. Details matter, and there is a certain 'feel' to a place. Those who have worked in several hospices say that there are different emphases, various atmospheres, that some are quieter or noisier than others, but with all the variations, there is a sense of imaginative care common to the hospice movement.

All hospitals have volunteer helpers, often in cafeterias and shops, but usually their numbers are limited. Hospices have specialized in the use of a wide range of voluntary helpers, usually co-ordinated by a member of staff. These services have grown naturally out of the charitable ethos of hospice origins. In the earliest days all was done without pay. A recently published history of St Barnabas' Hospice in Worthing recounts how both the first Medical Director and the first Matron came out of retirement and worked voluntarily for a number of years. Gradually the volunteer service has evolved from being a fairly haphazard group of those who wished the place well (and occasionally those who sought a social cachet from their association with such a prestigious place) to a highly organized venture, with rigorous interviews, contracts, a system of accountability, training courses and long-service awards. Salaried Co-ordinators and Secretaries have been appointed. Not all volunteers from the early days have appreciated the need for such organization, and the attitude that claims special treatment because 'I'm doing you a favour' can lead to tensions and resignations. Not all who volunteer are suitable for work in a hospice, and many sore hearts and hurt egos have had to be comforted, occasionally by the chaplain. There was a fear that 'ghouls', people with an unnatural interest in death, would volunteer although that fear seems to have been misplaced. There have been a number of unbalanced people and those working out their own bereavement problems, but with the professionalization of the hospice has come more control and no lessening of the number of willing people. Because Edinburgh has a relatively large number of professional persons, many of the first volunteers were those who had leisure, no need to work, and wonderful accents. As more and more relatives and friends of patients join the ranks, the volunteers reflect a more balanced cross-section of the community.

Volunteers serve in many ways, as drivers, flower-arrangers, ward-helpers, receptionists, fund-raisers, and gardeners. Many serve in the charity shops, others in the cafeterias, a few as nurses, and some in the chaplaincy team. There are bound to be difficulties with a 'mixed economy' of salaried and unsalaried staff, and there can be resentments over recognition and status, but the community of professionals and volunteers working together not only eases the financial burden, but adds to the atmosphere of home, and of hospitality, and gives a sense of connectedness to the local community. A strong volunteer group enables the immediate local community to feel some ownership of its hospice.

All homes have neighbours, and at a time when the NIMBY (not in my back yard) attitude is common, it is not surprising that not all of them were happy to find that a hospice was being opened on their doorsteps. For one thing, visitors and professionals mean cars and cars have to be parked. Then there was the question of hearses. Would a pleasant area be invaded by black cars? And some folk simply did not relish the thought of so much death near their homes. When an HIV/AIDS hospice was set up in the city there were even more complaints from neighbours. We hope that prejudices have been overcome, and so long as cars are courteously parked harmony has been achieved, and indeed many neighbours are volunteers and friends. This all adds to the feeling of the unit being 'home' rather than 'a home'.

While a single person can make a home, the concept usually implies family, young and old, women and men together in various relationships. If the hospice is in any way to resemble home it will reflect this. It has been suggested that the Medical Director is Father and the Nursing Director, especially if she, or he, is Matron, is Mother. The Administrative Director is described as a visiting aunt or uncle, and no doubt the Chaplain could be the local minister, perhaps a memory from childhood.[7] This may be a little fanciful, but parentlike attributes are given to the perceived leaders. Certainly there is a co-operation between men and women, and there are many more women than men on hospice staffs. It is not without significance that the founder of the modern hospice movement is Dame Cicely Saunders, and that women continue to play their part in leadership as administrators, doctors and chaplains, not only in the traditional female roles of nurses and flower-arrangers. There are some male nurses, and many male volunteers who serve tea, are hairdressers, and occasionally arrange flowers, as well as fulfilling the traditional male roles of drivers, fund-raisers and gardeners. It has been remarked that hospices have a feminine character, and this may be because women have a special aptitude for caring for the dying, or it may simply be that the greater number of staff are nurses and palliative care has yet to attract many male nurses.

When one is at home, one relaxes, puts on slippers and sits in the favourite armchair. At least this is a popular image. More realistically, home is where one is known, accepted, cared for, cosseted and shouted at, loved and corrected. Home is a safe place, where pretence is stripped away. To be at home is to be surrounded with familiar things and people, it is to be accepted with all the faults and virtues that make up a person. It is not to be alone, and it is to be safe. If a hospice offered all this it would be negating one of its purposes, which is to encourage sick people to live in their own home for as long as they can, and yet folk must be made to feel as much at ease in the hospice as possible. There is a sense of informality, reflected in the use of familiar names, which sometimes surprises visitors.

Sir Archibald had been a colonial governor, and was now a tired old man who responded warmly to the care of the staff. He told them that his name was Archie, and thus he was addressed, to his delight. Then a visiting cousin overheard and complained to the Governors that a patient was being insulted by 'youngsters' who did not treat him with the respect to which he was accustomed. A little negotiation was needed to reassure the relative. Once we looked after a titled gentleman who liked to be called Jock. I was amused to hear his son asking the volunteer receptionist if he could visit the Marquis of X and being told there was no one of that name on the list! Naming is important, for to some extent our name defines who we are, and how we appear to others. Among the staff there is a free use of given names, and every patient is asked how they would like to be addressed. Occasionally we entertain a 'Mrs' or a 'Miss,' or even a 'Doctor', but usually familiar names are used without offence or loss of dignity. Boundaries are necessary, and it is not wise to overstep them.

There has been a general loosening of formality in society, and on the whole, if this is not misused, it has been a good thing, another factor in making the patient feel at home. A modified familiarity, which does not forget dignity and privacy, can be practised.

Just as the hospice should have some aspects of a family, so the real family of the patient is of utmost importance. Jenny had nursed her husband of 57 years, who had prostate cancer, for as long as she could. She was exhausted, and had not slept properly for weeks. 'I lie at night with one ear open,' she said. She had promised Tom that she would keep him at home. He had had enough of radiotherapy, and he disliked hospitals, and as for the hospice, that was the place he least wanted to be, although he had a good relationship with the Home Care sister. But inevitably the day came when Jenny's doctor and the Home Care sister insisted that for her sake Tom must come to the hospice. Guiltily she allowed him to be taken there – 'taken away' was how she put it – and soon a volunteer driver brought her in to see Tom. At first he was reproachful and her guilt increased. Day by day however he became more at ease, and Jenny began to get a little rest. She shyly approached the sister one day, asking if she could share Tom's care, and help with feeding him. Their long close relationship was partly restored, she felt less guilty, and found satisfaction in washing his face and spooning in his porridge. The nurses had to adjust to allowing some of the care to be taken out of their professional hands, but they soon realized the necessity of this.

Of course a hospice can never be home. Home is where we live and relax, where we are most intimate and where we can entertain others. It may have been the natural place for death to occur, but that is no longer true. A hospice is always a sub-stitute, attempting to relieve anxiety, to give comfort and companionship, but by its very nature it can never be called a real home.

But it should be homelike, welcoming, relaxed yet highly professional, warm and friendly. There are evidently limits on its use as home. Other patients have to be taken into con-sideration. David and Connie had argued and fought all their married life. They were not quiet or restful folk. They seemed fond enough of each other, but when David came in to visit after being in the pub, there were scenes. What could we do? Other families were complaining, and so were the nurses. A single room did not seem to be the solution. Noises could still pour out from it. Eventually a senior doctor had a firm word with David, whose reaction was surprisingly mild. He had not realized how much of a nuisance he and Connie were making of themselves, and as he gradually absorbed the atmosphere, his behaviour changed. His fear of the place abated and he did not need to drink before he came in. This was a mild form of behaviour modification, and it worked – at least for the other patients and staff. It could of course be suggested that the respectability of middle-class expectations made David and Connie's conduct less authentically their own.

Indeed the clean and decent surroundings can cause discomfort. For whose benefit is the neglected old man, who has been living alone in an untended house for years, washed, shaved and generally brushed up? And when the tea lady comes with china cups and sugar lumps, is it surprising that he looks uncomfortable? Homelike behaviour is encouraged, but only when it does not transgress the norms of hospice etiquette. It is disconcerting when two sons of a patient choose the reception area for one of their regular fights or when two estranged daughters begin to shout at each other over their mother's bed. These tensions will continue, as will the attempt to make people feel at home.

One of the greatest dangers that hospice staff encounter is that of extravagant praise. We are sometimes told that nurses are all angels, that doctors are so unbelievably kind, and that the place is like a 'five star hotel', which is an eccentric definition of home! Sometimes it seems we do what we set out to do too well. When, as happens occasionally, there are complaints about the food, or the beds, or the conduct of the nurses, we tend to be taken aback. Dealing with patients who do not like us, men who will not speak to a woman doctor, or to someone who 'does not speak proper English', or relatives who have a litigious edge to their conversation, brings out the worst in us.

The care of the family is not a task to be lightly undertaken. There may be one significant person, or scores. Many people are content to believe that doctor knows best and some try hard not to have any encounters with staff. Others require an update each day or even more often, and are seen with note-book in hand, recording all the information they receive and the questions they still want to ask, and in many families there seems to be an alarming lack of communication. Family members in other countries use the telephone and e-mail, and sometimes the long-lost son arrives from Australia or the United States full of guilt at his neglect, guilt that shows itself in criticism of everything in the old country, especially its medical care. Often families are much less ready to accept the inevitability of the patient's death than the patient herself.

Mark knew that he was very ill. He had no energy and, thanks to the ministrations of the staff, minimal discomfort. He just wanted, at 82, to slip away, not to waken in the morn-ing. But Mark's daughters thought differently. They could not accept that their father was dying, and they spent, all four of them, hours at his bedside, shaking him awake, talking loudly among themselves, trying to make Mark eat, when he had no appetite and only wanted to be left in peace. When the nurses tried to persuade them to moderate their visits, or to go home for a few hours, they were met with anger and tears and accusations of cruelty. At last they all left the room for a few minutes, and Mark sighed and died. Strangely, the family was quite accepting after the first few minutes of anger and regret. I am sure that dying persons can be held in this world by their relatives and not allowed to die. Doctors can provide much anecdotal evidence for this. Patients can be seen to relax and let go when their families say goodbye. On the other hand, like Mark's relatives, families can strengthen the patient's ability to live, even when the will has gone. This is one of the many mysterious areas at the boundaries of life and death. Part of the hospice's task is to help relatives to come to terms with reality and to give the dying permission to get on with their death.

Not all families or units of cohabitation follow traditional lines. Many couples, at different stages of life, live together without formal marriage ceremony. More complicated arrangements can be encountered, and call for a suspension of judgement and an understanding acceptance by hospice staff. Same-sex couples are also in need of hospice care, and help can be given to reconcile parents and to allow open disclosure of sexual preferences and allegiances. The experience of AIDS hospices must be of help to the more general units in this area, fraught as it is with prejudice and changing social mores.

Children have their own special needs. Young children (usually, but not always, grandchildren and great-grandchildren of patients) seem to be happy to visit, to play with the toys we provide, and sometimes to go off to visit other grannies. The very young do not seem to have much fear of people who are in bed or obviously ill and tiny babies make their own special contributions. But as children grow older, and become more questioning about life and death, or reach a very shy stage, they may refuse to come, or they may have many questions that their parents do not feel competent to answer. Teenaged children of young patients often need to be taken aside by experienced staff, and receive explanations for the physical changes in their parent. Some children are very calm and accepting of the approach of death, and some have been caring for mother or father at home for some time, or may never remember a fit parent. Others have been shielded by their families, and need to be told in the right way, perhaps several times, just what is happening.

Two quite opposite reactions to the suggestion that young children might attend a funeral have impressed me. One group of parents simply assumes that this is normal; the other group is horrified. A few seek advice, and we have learnt that it is often the grandparents, who have grown up after the second world war, and who are the first generation to accept the so-called privatization of death, who are the most reluctant to let the children know the reality, and face the funeral.

Families extend beyond people. 'Pets may be admitted, so long as they are well-behaved.' Such is the regulation in the booklet families are given. There are many stories told about pets in a hospice and for some patients the welfare of dog or cat is a great worry, and a visit from the dog is reassuring. Cats are less able to visit, although some have been brought in special containers. But dogs enjoy coming, and for those patients to whom they have been constant companions they are a stimulus and a theme in subsequent conversation. Trained 'therapets', often retired guide dogs, visit and are welcomed, and patients who will scarcely speak to staff have been known to talk to a visiting dog. Phoebe was totally silent, an old woman about whom we knew little, lost in her own secret world. When the associate chaplain brought his new Labrador puppy in, she began to speak, until it was quite difficult to stop her. 'There are more germs on your shoes than on the dog's paws,' the medical director told a visitor outraged at the sight of a visiting dog.

A hospice can never be home, however hard patients, family and staff try, but it can be homelike, and it can be and usually is welcoming and reassuring. It will always be a place of mystery, and even those who have heard little of it associate it with death and therefore with darkness and gloom. People are pleasantly surprised by light and brightness, laughter and friendliness, but many will always remain wary and homesick.

For some, it will always be just another hospital, another place where they are fed at set times, and where they are cared for by folk in uniforms. Medicines, injections, baths performed in new ways, with hoists and with someone present, regulated visiting hours, and the presence of other sick people make it seem unreal to talk of being like home. There are patients who cannot leave soon enough, and some who discharge themselves. There are families who are quite prepared, indeed anxious to take their loved one home to die, and that can be arranged, even on the last day of life.

There are others who are so much at home in the hospice that they are reluctant to go back to their real home. 'Settling in' can pose a real problem. It is possible to set a time limit to admission – two weeks, and then the patient must go somewhere else. But somehow there are those who can avoid that. Families are relieved when Granny is admitted to the hospice. They will not have to care for her any longer, and they are assiduous visitors, only vanishing when a doctor approaches to discuss a return home for the old lady, who is much better with a little warmth and an adjustment of medication. Since not all patients deteriorate as expected, and a few seem to begin to recover, the staff is faced with quite hard choices. The hospice is not designed for long-stay patients. It is not easy for most people to see the next bed vacated more than once. It seems dangerous to make friends if yet another friend is going to die. So we encourage people to go home, and about 40 per cent do, according to recent statistics. This is quite an increase on early years, and quite contrary to the still common perception of a hospice as a place which you 'only leave in a box'. 'You come in the front door and go out the back door,' I was told recently.

There may be no one at home, and the house itself might be quite unsuitable, with awkward stairs and an inaccessible toilet. Occupational therapists, community nurses and home helps can do much, but without the co-operation of family and neighbours, it is sometimes impossible to contemplate sending a patient home. Occasionally the relatives have already given the keys back to the housing department or cleared or even sold the house, on the assumption that hospice implies imminent death. Then other accommodation must be sought. Nursing homes have proliferated in recent years, but finance can be a problem. Occasionally a family is quite open about the advantages of keeping Granny in the hospice where there are no charges, unless they wish to contribute, whereas the hoped-for legacy might vanish into nursing home fees. This is an area where rapid changes in our care of the elderly and sick are having an impact.

Of course the hospice can never be a real home, of course patients will long to go back to the familiar things, even for a quick visit. To pretend otherwise would be to delude our patients and ourselves. But photographs on the locker, little treats brought in by family, and the continued sense of sharing in the family life can make a stay there more tolerable. The very scale of the place helps to make it more homelike, and the *hospitium* offered and received enrich many who live and work in it.

FOR FURTHER THOUGHT

1 Can or should a hospice resemble a home?
2 How can a hospice be welcoming to a wide variety of people without losing its character?

NOTES

1 Cf. 3 John, Romans 16 and the Didache, among many other texts.
2 Jennifer Hockey, *Experiences of Death: an Anthropological Account.* Edinburgh: Edinburgh University Press 1990, pp. 168–9.
3 Katherine Froggatt, 'Rites of passage and the hospice culture' in *Mortality* 2:3 (July 1997), pp. 123–36.
4 *Op. cit.*, p. 125.
5 *Op. cit.*, p. 131.
6 Julia Lawton, *The Dying Process: Patients' Experiences of Palliative Care.* London: Routledge 2000, pp. 168–9.
7 This analogy is set out in D. Graves, 'Models of hospice management' in *Hospice Management* (factsheet 9) published by St Christopher's Hospice.

CHAPTER FIVE

The Hospice as School

When the Hospice of St James, Anytown, which we have already visited, was founded, it was perceived in the eyes of many early supporters as a quiet monastic institution where the dying could live out their last days in peace and quiet. These were quite early days of hospice development, when the work of enthusiastic professionals had not acquired its own academic standing, and when consultants at local hospitals could dismiss the hospice as a place run by general practitioners and volunteers. When the vision of the hospices as a place of learning, study and research began to be promoted there was heated argument, and indeed considerable conflict, involving the founding mothers and fathers and the directors whom they had chosen. The founding group had sacrificed money, time and indeed reputation to promote their vision of a peaceful retreat. The newly appointed medical director had quite a different vision. She foresaw a much more professional institution, with its doors open to students and researchers, and with her eye on national and even international regard. There were long and painful tussles before the idea began to be accepted.

Today it seems obvious that a hospice, while it has as its primary purpose the care of very sick people and their families, is also a place where students from various disciplines can learn about the care of the dying, and can discover skills to take into the wider world. What was envisaged as being a quiet retreat has become a busy academy. The image of the doctor, surrounded by his penumbra of (usually) eager students, standing at the foot of the bed and discussing the patient without asking more than a token permission, seemed far from the hospice ideal. Many safeguards needed to be put in place to preserve privacy and dignity for the patients.

Yet, within the first few months, as we discovered in Edinburgh, medical students and eager general practitioners began to appear from far and near, anxious to know what this new thing was. The medical director summoned a conference of local clergy, limited to twenty persons, and sixty applied. So several day courses were laid on. The Faculty of Divinity at the University and other theological colleges and seminaries began to send students for placement, and almost imperceptibly the hospice became a place of education. Social workers, home helps, physiotherapists and many other professionals followed, and gradually a very full programme of nurse education, now achieving degree status, evolved.

All this could not happen without opposition. It was stressed that patients should not be seen as objects of professional interest and investigation. Access to the wards has always been jealously guarded. Occasionally families expressed concern that those they care about are being used or disturbed, but patients, assigned to meet medical students, are often delighted to be of use, and can be heard boasting that they had been lecturing to future doctors. The concept of the hospice as a place of education has at length been accepted and the building of a lecture hall and ancillary seminar rooms and then a whole suite of offices for Nurse-Lecturers made this evident.

Alongside such physical developments, which are commonplace in hospices throughout the United Kingdom, came the development of specialist education. Palliative medicine, which seemed to be a poor relation of oncology or geriatrics, became a specialist discipline in the1980s, and is now said to be one of the largest specialisms in medicine in the UK. Training posts were created, with funding from the Macmillan Fund and other sources. Chairs of Palliative Medicine were set up in London and Alberta, Canada, and subsequently in several other universities. Hospice doctors, instead of being dismissed as enthusiasts with peculiar tastes and missionary zeal, were perceived as belonging to mainstream medicine. Registrars applied for jobs as consultants, consultants became medical directors, and a whole new hierarchy was born, under the watchful eyes of Post-Graduate Deans. And this happened very quickly. Now doctors can choose to spend most of their careers in palliative medicine, and as specialists they are required to become involved in research projects. Journals such as *Palliative Medicine* and the *European Journal of Palliative Care* were launched and soon became established. Articles and reports, books and reviews, films and videos seemed to pour from the presses.

While medical and nursing training has contained much clinical information and pharmacological content, the inclusive nature of hospice care had made it inevitable that training in psychological and spiritual aspects of the dying has occupied a prominent place. Young medical students, who can find that lectures and workshops on communication skills are not necessarily what they are looking for in a clinical environment, have not always appreciated this. All they want is information on pain-relief techniques and medical matters. Some theological students have failed to see the relevance of specialized pastoral care to their ministry of preaching and discipline. Nurses have been put off by the words 'spiritual care' which they tend to equate with religious zeal. But courses have usually been favourably assessed, and teaching staffs at sending institutions have become very enthusiastic about the impact of hospice ideas on their students.

In the area of nurse training, specialist palliative-care nurse teachers emerged in the 70s and 80s, and it was found that many nurses, from within the hospices and from general hospitals, nursing homes and the community were anxious to improve their understanding and skills. Some were willing to finance themselves, if necessary, to attend courses, which, in Edinburgh, developed into a BSc degree in Palliative Nursing. It became obvious that all nurses, trained or auxiliary, should undergo in-service training. Recently, the Bridges Project, designed to bring the insights of palliative care into nursing homes, and to learn from them the difficulties and the particular culture of institutions caring for the elderly, has been instituted, as a research project. It has been recognized that in Edinburgh at least the number of folk dying in nursing

homes has increased rapidly in recent years, following the clo-
sure of many NHS geriatric wards and the opening of more
long-stay homes.

Clergy and students for the ministry form two of the target
groups in hospice education and the process is sufficiently
mature to allow some assessment to be made. Since about
1970 the teaching of pastoral or practical theology has been
transformed. No longer does it only supply 'hints and tips' for
practitioners, and assume that most caring skills will be learnt
from a more senior minister or by doing the job. No longer is
it simply seen as an appendage to 'real' theology. There is
much more emphasis on monitored placements, contact with
caring institutions, and on theological and personal reflection. Pastoral or practical theology has fought for its position
in syllabuses and in the general field of theological education.
The growing hospice movement has been well placed to take
advantage of these developing ways of training. Most theological colleges and seminaries in the UK make some provision
for teaching ordinands about death, dying and bereavement,
and lecturers from hospices and specialist palliative care
units have taken part in such programmes. Some colleges set
apart a teaching week for the subject and include sociological
and anthropological background, and such practical matters
as visits to crematoria and discussions with undertakers.
Others seem to concentrate more on theology, liturgy and
the tradition of the churches. Various methods are in use, and
the whole subject is now treated as important in the training
of clergy. The ability to deal with the dying is no longer seen
as being bestowed by ordination alone, as it once was.

DAY COURSES

Colleges of all shades of theological opinion appear to find a
hospice a useful and even comfortable place to send students
for a day course. Typically there will be an introduction to the
ethos of the hospice, and lectures from a doctor, a Home Care
sister, and the chaplains, with time for lively discussion, and
a session on bereavement issues. Teaching on the site has many
advantages, and students are willing to travel some distance

to share in this. Access to patients and the Day Hospice is not permitted but it would be impossible not to be aware of what is going on in the wards. Over the years students from Roman Catholic, Episcopalian, Free Church of Scotland and Baptist Colleges have spent fruitful days catching a glimpse of hospice life. Much more mixed groups from the university faculties of Divinity have included candidates for the ministry of the Church of Scotland, and many others studying practical theology for a great variety of reasons. In recent years the group from St Mary's College, the Theology Faculty of the University of St Andrews, has been made up of a mixture of theology and medical students who are studying a module on pastoral care. Evaluations have usually been very positive, and the questions raised have stimulated the chaplains, and no doubt the other lecturers. Occasionally the hospice has been seen as irrelevant to 'real' ministry, and has been accused of palliating real spiritual needs. 'Do you confront your patients with the possibility of hell?' is a question designed to upset hospice chaplains. The image of a cosy middle-class enclave is hard to dispel, as is the urge in some theology students to witness to their faith vocally and to attempt to rescue sinners on the brink of death. These matters arise in discussion, and are sometimes reflected in evaluation by those too polite to speak while on the visit, but when students come on placement, from whatever background, the theological difficulties seem to be quickly resolved when real people are encountered. Philip knew, when he came to spend a few days at the hospice, that his section of the Church was *the* Church. It alone held the whole truth. Others were sadly mistaken, and he was prepared to make allowances for environment and lack of proper teaching. But he was confronted by Molly, who belonged to quite a different tradition. He was Anglo-Catholic, she was Free Church of Scotland. When they met, they immediately found common ground in their love for animals. From that shared interest they progressed to speaking about their perceptions of faith and then to praying together. It was impossible to tell who gained the most from the brief friendship. Real ecumenical discussion often bypasses the committees and conferences we set up.

Day courses for ordained clergy have followed a similar pattern, and those who attend are self-selected. The initial enthusiasm to attend has diminished as more have become familiar with the hospice movement and many have already been introduced to it as students. Not only ordinands and clergy have taken advantage of hospice training. Groups of pastoral visitors, elders, and bereavement care teams from local churches have spent time with us, and there has been considerable input into lay training schemes of various churches.

PLACEMENTS

Over the years colleges have offered a placement at a hospice as an option for clergy in training. Practices vary, but the aim of allowing a student to learn under supervision and to reflect on what is learned has been central. Students may attend once a week for one or more terms. They may come for a one-week block, and some, especially those from other countries, have become assistant chaplains for a considerable number of hours each week. Because a hospice is usually a small unit, there is not space for many students at one time, nor is there occupation for many hours each day, so various possibilities have to be considered. One of the problems that the chaplain faces in organizing placements and courses is that different branches of the Christian Church (and, so far, only Christians have shown an interest in such training although those of other faith communities may well do so in future) have different expectations of their students. The formation of a Free Church of Scotland minister is not the same as that of a Roman Catholic priest. Traditions differ within denominations, and there can be no uniform pattern. When teaching on reflective practice was given at a recent course, several of the students said that they had become jaded with the process, while some others, from a quite different kind of college, had never heard of it. In this disparity theological education is distinct from medical or nursing training. It is much more untidy, and such research as has been undertaken into provision of courses in the care of the dying in training institutions gives only an outline pattern of expectations and resources.

Nevertheless students from diverse traditions have reacted to actual patient contact in remarkably similar ways. Nursing staff have occasionally expressed a fear that theology students will try to proselytize, but in my experience this has not been a problem. A gentle pastoral approach, and a desire to learn from those visited and their families has been common. A student working with the City Mission caused apprehension because of the understanding the staff, and indeed the chaplain, had of that institution. One day the student sighed and said, 'It's wonderful not to have to evangelize all the time!'

Some years ago two students from the theological college of the Scottish Episcopal Church were placed at St Columba's Hospice on Wednesday afternoons. Subsequently they wrote of their experiences and their reflections were published as prize essays in *Contact*.[1] They wrote of their fears of approaching dying persons. Conscious of being identified as theological students they expected to be questioned about their own beliefs about death, aware of their uncertainties, and doubtful about their ability to be companions on the journey that patients were engaged in. One writes of his feelings of uselessness and illegitimacy, and on the paradox of faith absent and present in himself as he met patients. Both discovered that the 'dying' were actually the living, and both also felt something of the cost of caring. One wrote:

> And so it was an occasion of sitting beside someone who most of the time could only sleep, which made the deepest impression on me ... suffering cancer had burned his faith, though only last week he'd talked astonishingly about Jesus' love for us, and of his own dying as heading for a white dot at the apex of a triangle ... His breathing was so shallow. Sometimes I feared he might die. And then it occurred to me, at the Hospice it is the dying who are visiting me. They are showing me something of the mystery of death, and healing memories of people I have known who have died. Their dying is helping me to live.[2]

They were both struck by a sense of God's presence even as they felt empty and useless.

These two students were particularly articulate, and they were expressing what many working in hospices have experienced. There is a special quality of love given and received in caring for the dying. Many students have commented on real changes taking place in their understanding of pastoral care in these surroundings, and have later claimed that the hospice experience has had a profound effect on their subsequent ministry. Others have seen their placement as one among several interesting experiences, but I believe that hospices offer an important training ground, and place of self-discovery for many women and men preparing for service in the church.

PRACTICAL WORK

Very early in our story a divinity student offered to spend one morning a week as a volunteer gardener. In these relatively unstructured days, this proved for him an excellent way to learn about the place, meet the staff, and sometimes patients. We had already begun to hold morning prayers and one morning he conducted them in his muddy gardening clothes and boots. This may seem a trivial incident, but for him it was an important point in ministerial formation. From time to time students from various colleges and seminaries have worked as auxiliary nurses, and for several years Jesuit novices were seen in uniform on the wards. For some of them it was the first time that they had worked in an institution that did not belong solely to their church, and for at least one young man it was a new experience to work alongside women.

Several hospices have conducted courses in which ward work has been integrated with study and lecture periods, and others have interdisciplinary courses, which include practical work, and in which students from very different backgrounds and with different career hopes have learned from one another.

LONGER COURSES

For many years there has been a longer course for senior theology students at St Columba's Hospice. It began when Anglican Colleges in the United Kingdom required that each student should complete two Pastoral Studies Units, whose length and other conditions were carefully specified. These were located in pastoral care situations outside normal church life. We were able to offer a course which met Anglican criteria, and extend it to students from other churches.

The Chaplain and the Nurse Tutor drew up the course, which for many years lasted for 13 teaching days and now consists of a more intensive ten. In 1982 we sent out our first intimation to theological colleges, and that year we accepted five. Since then there have been six or seven each autumn, and in 2000 fifteen students from such varied colleges as the College of the Resurrection (Anglo-Catholic and monastic), the Free Church of Scotland College in Edinburgh (Presbyterian and conservative), New College, Edinburgh (Church of Scotland and many others), Oak Hill Church of England College, London, the various federated colleges in Manchester, Regents Park Baptist College, Oxford, and the former Gillis Roman Catholic Seminary, Edinburgh. For several years we have welcomed as guests on the course students from the Metropolitan Seminary of the Catholic Church in Krakow, Poland, as a small contribution to the work of the hospice movement in that country. We have had Scottish, English, Danish, Polish, Chinese and Peruvian students on the course, and the interplay between people of different denominational backgrounds and different traditions within churches has been fascinating to share.

The aims of the course are:

1 The acquiring of information about all aspects of palliative care, involving the study of the problems of patients and relatives, medical, social, emotional and spiritual;

2 The development of practical and theological skills, including the ability to form relationships with dying patients and their families, some skills in communication, and an appreciation of the possibilities of inter-disciplinary co-operation;

3 Personal reflection leading to growth, stressing the ability to integrate experience into a developing theological understanding of life, death and the gospel.

The basic structure of the course is a series of lectures on aspects of human development, self-understanding, and communication, interspersed with an introduction to cancer care, a discussion of the theology of death and dying, and a study of the emotional and spiritual needs of patients families and carers. Because it is part of our purpose to remind students that most people do not die in hospices, we have visits from a geriatrician, a chaplain to a general hospital and someone involved with the care of dying children. Our friendly undertaker adds a different dimension, and we have included from time to time lectures on the needs of ethnic communities, on organ transplants, and the AIDS hospice, and always we have a longer session on the ethical question raised by palliative care.

Integral to the course are daily acts of worship with the students taking turns to conduct the regular morning prayers for patients, volunteers and staff. At the end of the course a variety of closing acts of worship has been devised, as we discovered that sometimes a eucharistic celebration could be more divisive than uniting. The course allows time for participants to talk together, and to learn about each other's traditions as well as to discuss the particular subject matter.

Access to patients has been a difficult issue. While one of the objects of the course has been to learn directly from the 'living human document', this has not been easy in practice. Those patients who are alert enough and agreeable to see students are often not available when the students are free. They may be entertaining visitors, or attending the Day Hospice, or waiting for lunch. So after years when there were times of frustration for students, and some unhappiness being expressed by the nursing staff at the prospect of six or more extra persons on the wards in the late morning, a new scheme was introduced whereby each student was able to meet one patient each week, and also to interview one member of staff and one volunteer, allowed the participants to gain a wider view of hospice life, and some understanding of the motivation of those who worked there. The obligatory case study, whose contents had hitherto been restricted to patients, could now be spread over a wider area of concern, and has developed into a reflective exercise.

Close contact with the hospice community teaches many lessons, some more obvious than others. Students have had to learn to accept rejection by sleepy or confused patients. Clergy do not like to be turned away as useless! One was very angry when 'his' patient had the effrontery to die suddenly before he had finished his case study. Another, a former officer in the Forces, was accused by a confused man who had been in ranks of refusing to let him go home. 'I have never been spoken to like that,' he said, with some bafflement and indignation. A doctor explained that the choice of student for blame was fairly random. Someone had to be held responsible for what the patient saw as an injustice, and hopefully the student is a better minister because of that episode.

A hospice is an enclosed community and pastoral students find themselves carefully observed not only by patients, but also by staff. Sometimes they behave like all theological students, laugh, argue, tell loud stories and generally make a noise. Conventional folk and older Edinburgh ladies among the staff and volunteers express surprise. Their stereotypes of the clergy have been shattered.

Two features of the course have become very important. Each student is assigned to a supervisor, often from outside the hospice, who meets with her at the beginning, in the middle and at the end of the course for confidential conversation. This has been of great benefit to the students, who have been able to reflect on what is happening to them during the course, and also to relate their learning to their own life-situations. An important place is also given to appraisal, and it is then, in the evaluation session at the end of the course, that out of the extravagant praise that we almost expect as hospice workers, emerge the frustrations and sometimes the anger of people on the threshold of their ministerial lives. We hope that we have learnt from the reactions and reformed our course in the light of what we have heard.

We have been careful in our selection and at first we were not happy about receiving any applicant who had had a recent bereavement. Experience has taught that students come with their own agenda. One student, despite the fears and indeed the prohibitions of the medical and nursing staff, found his way into a room to speak with a young male patient. It was the very room in which the student's brother, also a young man, had died two years previously. The student found this a profoundly helpful, if difficult, experience.

There are obvious disadvantages in a course for only one discipline, and interdisciplinary courses have a special value. Nevertheless I have found the annual invasion hard to organize, but challenging and rewarding, and we take comfort in the fact that certain colleges send us students every year.

The hospice is also a school for all who work in it. We hope we learn a little about the care of the dying. We certainly discover a great deal about human nature and about ourselves. It is our hope that those in all caring disciplines who spend some time with us will take what they learn and apply it in their work, and that all those who make use of the services will discover something of value and meaning in what they encounter.

FOR FURTHER THOUGHT

1 Was it a wise move for hospices to become involved in teaching?
2 How can lessons learnt be integrated in the wider life of the hospital and the church?

NOTES

1 I. Barcroft and D. Broad in *Contact* 93:2 (1987), pp. 26–30.
2 *Op. cit.*, p. 29.

CHAPTER SIX

The Hospice as Laboratory

Because a hospice is a small and specialized unit it is a good place in which to examine questions which have a much wider reference. In all caring institutions decision-making and information-sharing are important issues, but because there is such a concentration of staff, and because of the relatively acute nature of the condition of many patients, in a hospice such issues are sharpened and clarified. It would not be proper to describe the hospice as a laboratory without making several qualifications. Patient welfare and privacy are paramount, and research and teaching must honour this. If the choice is between gathering evidence for a research paper, and allowing the patient to enjoy her chosen silence when questioned, then the patient's wishes must come first. Tender loving care and laboratory conditions do not seem to go together. Yet it is inevitable that there will be experiments, whether with drugs, dressings, or with forms of liturgy and inter-church co-operation, in which patients will be involved, knowingly or not.

ETHICAL ISSUES

Euthanasia will be considered in Chapter Seven. It is the most obvious ethical issue in hospice care, and the one students most often ask us about, but there are several other ethical questions which arise at the end of life. Sarah is a young woman in St James Hospice, Anytown, who has motor neurone disease. She can no longer walk, and she travels by electric wheelchair. She has limited use of her hands, and her speech is very indistinct. She is able to use an electronic device to

communicate. Until recently we were told that MND in its
most usual, though still mercifully uncommon, form had a
timescale of two years from diagnosis to death. With new
feeding and other techniques patients now can live much
longer. Sarah does not seem to have deteriorated much over
the last few months. She occupies the most spacious single
room, entertains her friends, and usually, but not always,
she co-operates with the nurses and the other patients. Not
surprisingly she sometimes becomes frustrated and angry at
her condition and takes her anger out on others. An electric
wheelchair can be an alarming weapon. Attempts to send her
home are blocked by her powerful sister, previously her main
carer, who fears she will not cope and threatens to go to the
press if Sarah is moved from St James. So efforts to find her
alternative care are constantly blocked. As Sarah cannot speak
her sister insists on speaking for her. Yet she does not seem to
be dying and she is using a bed and other valuable resources.
What is the duty of the hospice? Despite the involvement of
social workers, and a specialist MND nurse, nothing appears
to be happening. Some resentment is growing among the
nurses. Doctors are frustrated. Yet we must go on caring.
Sarah's case is a fairly extreme example of a not uncommon
ethical dilemma. What do we do with the patient who is not
imminently dying? Elderly folk may be as likely to die of old
age as of cancer. There is always the temptation for the
harassed GP or the busy consultant to see the hospice as a
refuge for a patient who is difficult to place.

Polly lived alone. She was a widow in her 70s, and she had
cancer. Her GP thought that the hospice was the right place for
her, as she had had radiotherapy and chemotherapy, and no
further treatment was indicated. She arrived and slept for the
better part of a week, and we called her nephew from afar.
The end seemed near. Then she woke up and began to eat,
and talk, and soon she was out of bed. She had few financial
resources, and the nephew was fairly distant and not too
keen to take responsibility for his aunt. But Polly's cancer
seemed to have gone into remission. With tempting food,
company and security – all good hospice offerings – she was
quite active, and began to take a great interest in other patients.

She considered herself indispensable in the ward, and was famously described by nurses as 'busybodying about'. Clearly she was not in the right place. Could she go home? That seemed unlikely, as she was quite unrealistic about her abilities to care for herself. Could she go to a nursing home? 'No,' said her nephew, 'no aunt of mine is going to one of those places. Wouldn't she have to pay, or would I?' Eventually, and with great reluctance, she did enter a nursing home and left the hospice in no kind mood. She felt rejected and unwanted, and her minister reported later that the transition to an excellent nursing home had led to a rapid decline in her condition. She gave up the struggle and died. Again the ethical question turned on the use of limited resources, and our duty to seek the patient's welfare. After all, she had not asked to come to the hospice. She had been sent, and good care had restored her to life for a time. There was quite a debate among doctors and nurses at the time on the morality of rejecting a patient, as it certainly seemed to her, and to the congregation to which she belonged, that such was the case. The local church certainly had expectations of the hospice which could not be fulfilled. The expectations of the church and the resources of the hospice no longer coincided.

As new treatments are discovered, tested and used, more people like Polly and Sarah will pose dilemmas. Should a hospice only welcome those in the last days of life? With the development of community and Day Hospice services, patients become involved in hospice care at earlier stages of illness. Multiple admissions to adjust medicines and to give carers respite are becoming common, and represent a very obvious change from earlier patterns, when many fewer patients returned home, even briefly.

THE PERCEPTION OF THE HOSPICE AS THE PLACE OF INEVITABLE DEATH

Certainly in the public mind the hospice is the last stage on the journey and families are often reluctant to allow patients to come in. All sorts of stories are told to patients by the well-meaning relatives. 'It's a nice nursing home, it's a convalescent hospital and we'll soon have you home.' Staff are occasionally ordered not to let the patient know where she is, an order somewhat difficult to carry out! There is still a fear that admission to a hospice is a death-sentence, and no amount of demonstration will convince some people that patients actually go home and have some quality of life.

A hospice should be a place of transparency and honesty, but it is difficult not to collude with the games that are being played both by relatives and by patients. How honest should staff be when questioned? There are many facets to this apparently simple question. It does not seem to be acceptable in many families to talk about a forthcoming death. Euphemisms abound, and hopes, often false, are encouraged. Vera knew she was dying. She was reluctant to die, as she would have loved to watch her grandchildren grow up, but as she remarked to the chaplain, 'I have had my three score years and ten, and we must all die.' This was not how her two daughters saw it. They apparently could not contemplate life without mother, and so they constantly spoke of her return to her own home, and of the holiday they would take her on very soon. When it was suggested that this was a very unlikely hope, they were angry, and refused to discuss Vera's illness with any professionals. As she grew weaker they were constantly leaning over the bed, trying to feed Vera, coaxing her to drink, not allowing her any peace, until suddenly the truth dawned on them and they became able to consider life without mother. Vera was peaceful from that day until a little while later, when she died. Not every family has a moment of truth like that.

Certainly there are times when the truth about dying must be faced. If the patient says 'Don't tell my husband – I know him and it will be too much for him to bear,' and the husband says the same about the patient, then skilful intervention is called for. But there are some people who have never been able to face unpleasant reality, and who will die in a state of what we like to call denial. It is hard not to apply our own norms to others and hard to give someone the freedom to believe and act in a way which we consider unhelpful, indeed untruthful. Yet not everyone wants a doctor who cheerfully announces the inevitability of death. To try to break a wall of denial can be cruel and benefit no one but the professional who is trying to carry out his expected role. And of course patients say different things to different carers, and try out one against another. All sorts of little games are played, consciously or otherwise.

PATIENT-CARER RELATIONSHIP

Perhaps in a bigger unit, or in the wider community, a doctor or nurse can have brief encounters with patients, then go off-duty, and never see the patient again. This is scarcely possible in the hospice. Because of the favourable staff-patient ratio, all relationships become more intense. Staff become attached to patients, and share the grief when they die. This grieving is cumulative. When we are asked if it is not depressing to work in such a place, we usually deny it, but sometimes we can confess to sadness, as so many people that we have known and been intimate with are no longer there and their place is taken by others. It would be unnatural if there did not grow up esteem and affection among staff, patients and families. It becomes dangerous only when one staff member appears to become too attached to a patient, and then others must give warnings, or the nurse or doctor must be transferred to work in another part of the unit. And sometimes hospice staff do find their work oppressive. They need an alternative world outside the gates.

Because cities are less impersonal than they are reputed to be, and are often simply collections of large villages, and because most of the staff will be local people, it is inevitable that from time to time friends and relatives will be admitted as patients. This may be an enriching experience, as loyal staff believe that they are giving good care to all their patients and so their aunt or cousin is in the best place. It can also be very reassuring for the patient, and add to the sense of familiarity and home, and it can sometimes be embarrassing. But it can also be disorienting. My older cousin Alex, to whom I had never been very close, was admitted with a brain tumour. Alex was an ex-army man, and we had always been a little wary of each other. His tastes and mine in language, humour and places to spend the evening did not quite coincide. But it was useful to have a minister in the family when it came to weddings and funerals. In the few days that he was in our ward I found myself looking at care with different eyes. This was my cousin, so why were his fingernails allowed to remain dirty? When his wife complained about the food – he was refusing to eat anything – I took it personally, as if I was the cook. When the sister reported that Alex had been rude to an auxiliary nurse during the night, I felt ashamed. It was a salutary experience to be a relative.

My lifelong friend Caroline, who was also a relative by marriage, came to us, alert, angry and articulate. She had been a missionary doctor for many years, and on her return to Scotland to care for her aged father had trained for the ministry of the Church. During her course she developed cancer, and by the time she graduated and was recognized by the church she was confined to a wheelchair, and then she deteriorated further, and came reluctantly to be looked after by 'these young doctors and nurses'. I fondly thought that I would be able to discuss with her the eternal dimensions of her predicament. She was, I knew, a realist, not frightened of speaking her mind, or of confronting her situation, and her strong faith was being tried in so many ways. She lost her appetite for food, and the only theological talk we had was on the significance of Jesus eating fish after the resurrection. 'Ghosts don't eat, so I'll be able to enjoy food in heaven,' she said. Then she discovered milkshakes and the wonderful uses of a naso-gastric tube, and one problem disappeared. What was more difficult was her frustration and anger, which she some-times vented on the doctors, who were all younger than she was. She occasionally appeared to doubt their skill, or spoke as if she did. I found that I was passing her room and hoping she was asleep, until I began to understand something of her dis-appointment, her anxiety about her father, and her frustration that she could not answer the call she had had to ministry.

CONFIDENTIALITY

When I was a less experienced minister I announced at our church prayer meeting that Mary, one of the older members who lived in an Eventide Home, had entered the Marie Curie Home in our county. I was summoned by the formidable Matron of the Eventide Home, and told that another church member had come and spread the news to the other residents. Very firmly I was told never again to mention Marie Curie or to imply that one of 'her' residents might have cancer. So I have been more careful since. Yet Mary was a believer in the power of prayer. She wanted her fellow church members to know what was happening. There is a real dilemma here. Other professionals, I am informed, often regard clergy as being notoriously unable to keep confidences. They want to tell the rest of the church community if someone is being admitted to a hospice. It seems unnatural to keep such a matter secret. On the other hand it is the patient's right whether or not to let his situation be known. Clergy are not privileged over others in sharing knowledge, nor have they visiting rights which override normal procedure. Patients may not want to see their minister at a particular moment, or they may be embarrassed by being in a hospice. They may have a very tenuous connection with the church and resent an intrusion into their privacy. There are many reasons why a minister must ask permission to visit. Occasionally the chaplain hears from a patient that she does not consider herself important enough for a visit from the minister, or that he must be too busy to give time to her, and then a little persuasion usually results in an important pastoral contact. If the patient believes in the power of prayer and the influence of the fellowship, it is sad if fellow believers are not allowed to share in care and pastoral prayer. But it is nevertheless the patient's right to be ashamed of having cancer, or of being so weak as to be ill.

Maisie was one of those missionaries who had overcome all obstacles to go to work in Africa. She had worked as a housemaid to raise enough money for her fare, and had managed to persuade a Faith Mission to adopt her as one of their staff. She had spent nearly forty years with few furloughs in her

chosen place of service in West Africa, and now in old age she
was admitted to the hospice with cancer. Nothing very sudden
was happening, and as I was brought up in the same church
and remembered her from when I was a boy, I suggested that
the Missionary Prayer Meeting should be informed of her illness. She was quite angry. 'You may tell them I have a heart
condition, not that I am here,' she said, and it was in vain that
I argued that she believed in prayer and had practised her
belief all her life. To her, as to other older people, cancer was
a 'dirty disease'. In time she went to an elderly persons' unit
in another hospital, and was then happy to receive visits and
let her frailty be mentioned.

RESEARCH INTO PRAYER AND THE
GOOD EFFECTS OF RELIGION

Despite attempts in recent years, research into the benefits of
faith and church-going have proved difficult to evaluate.
Anecdotal evidence suggests that some of those who seem to
have little faith in any conventional sense face impending
death with great equanimity, while others, who have made it
clear that they are believers, and are supported by fellow
believers, have found death too awful to face, or have been
angry that their faith has not exempted them from fatal illness.
Russell Stannard, in his book *The God Experiment*, describes
the Benson study into the effects of prayer on patients undergoing heart surgery.[1] Three groups of 600 patients are being
investigated. The first group are prayed for by special teams
of intercessors drawn from a variety of Christian denominations, but are unaware of this. Patients in the second group
will not be prayed for, and are the control group. The third
group will be told they are being prayed for, to find out if this
has a placebo or other effect. It is too early to know the results
yet, but if there is a statistically positive correlation between
prayer and good recovery from the operation then there is
scope for many follow-up investigations. It seems difficult to
be sure of any conclusions from this kind of experiment. What
about friends of those patients who are not being officially
prayed for? These friends might be very active in prayer, as

might be the patients themselves. The researchers refer to this as 'unwanted background noise'! Does it not seem that the experiment suggests that God can be somehow constrained to answer by healing, and not in other ways? The same objections can be raised against other such experiments, yet in a research-based culture, these attempts will continue to be made. Certainly patients who are well supported and obviously loved have a certain security that more isolated persons lack. This is an area which will impinge on hospice care, with interesting outcomes.

PALLIATIVE THEOLOGY

I must make my background clear. I was brought up in a family intimately connected with the leading evangelical congregation in Edinburgh. At least that is what we were always taught! We are rooted in a Revival movement, which took place parallel to, and influenced by, the Welsh Revival of 1904–5, and we know that we are different. When I was young, the church was, and still is, large, well attended, and to a certain extent endogamous, so that my family on both sides would be there on a Sunday and during the week. We hardly had need for friends in other Baptist churches, far less 'in the world'. At school there was a meeting of the Scripture Union,[2] to which I was allowed to go, but most other after-school activities were forbidden. Even when I went to university in Edinburgh I continued to live at home and only grudgingly was I allowed to attend the Christian Union. There was and is now in the church a lively, well run Scout group, with its own holiday centre on the coast, and an energetic Young People's meeting, where we learnt to reason, criticize and be loyal at the same time. The emphasis was on sharing our faith, witnessing and evangelizing, all of which I believed I should do, but found hard, as I was shy and did not want to be too different from my school friends. It was a secure, certain environment in which to grow up, and I am eternally grateful for it, and for the preaching I heard in my youth from two outstanding expositors. But looking back, I know that I imbibed a very strong sense that we were the chosen people, that everyone else was not only wrong but foolish not to see the Bible as we did, and that there was a firm, strong line to be drawn between the saved and the unsaved, and between those who would go to heaven, and those who would not. Our ministers were not afraid to speak of hell and the dangers of damnation. Nor were they slow to criticize the words and works of other forms of the Christian faith. And of course we were well informed about foreign missions and the evangelization of the heathen.

I have indulged in this autobiographical fragment because I think it is important that as chaplains we should know where we are in theological terms, and what baggage we carry with us into palliative care. I have been struck by how much ministers and priests of very different background have in common when they are in touch with the dying, and this is perhaps one aspect of palliative theology. Certain well discussed and indeed important barriers are dented and have gates inserted in them, or at least stiles built over them, and there is a cross-denominational dialogue, which is not so easy elsewhere. A mature candidate for the ministry with a military background told me that looking back, it was a visit to a hospice which had made the first serious challenge to his hitherto rigid perception of the ways of God.

But we are still shaped by our backgrounds, and there is no point in denying our convictions. For the last few years a number of students for the ministry of the Church of Scotland training at New College, Edinburgh, have been required to attend a Hospitals Week at the Edinburgh Royal Infirmary (general hospital) and the Royal Edinburgh Hospital (psychiatric hospital) and to spend a day at St Columba's Hospice. Some of them reported back to the college that the chaplains of these institutions had lost their evangelistic urge, and had become universalists. This rather unfair conclusion made us think and reflect on our position, and also wonder what sort of pastors the national church was training.

It is from this background that I want to think about a theology which is influenced by the palliative care movement. Shortly after my appointment as part-time chaplain at a hospice I was at a Baptist prayer meeting and heard a woman pray that I should rescue many brands from the burning. I felt an instant revulsion to this kind of 'turn or burn' theology, and I have been trying ever since to synthesize my experience and my evangelical upbringing.

Can anyone draw clear lines between the saved and the others in a hospice? It is said that one of our patients who himself was a minister had a notebook in which he entered the names of the staff under three categories – those who were Christians, those who thought they were and were deluded, and those who definitely were not. This may have been a true story, but fortunately it remains unique!

There are still Christians who profess to believe in hell, and certainly many who believe in a good afterlife, usually equated with heaven. But, as Walter points out in *The Eclipse of Eternity*, belief in the afterlife, or at least in a life after death affected by our behaviour and belief here, has become attenuated. Even in such an apparently dogmatic church as the Roman Catholic, there has been a softening, at least in practice, and David Lodge could say, in his novel about growing up in the 1960s *How Far Can You Go*, that hell died in that decade. When I read that book, I felt many resonances with my own upbringing, in what seemed a quite different milieu. What for most Christians was axiomatic certainly well into the Victorian era – despite *The Decline of Hell*, D. P. Walker's book in which he describes radical thinkers of the seventeenth century – has now become almost a curiosity, 'a statistically deviant belief'.[3] Even if preachers proclaim the fear of hell, they cannot assume that their hearers will accept and tremble. I have very seldom found a patient who volunteered a statement that suggested she was afraid of future punishment, although there have been a few who have expressed fear that they have not been good enough for God's approbation. In two papers, 'Spiritual Terrorism' and 'Spiritual Abuse', an American chaplain has described the impact of a form of fundamentalism on dying patients.[4] Although I could recognize the concepts and the language, the dangers they point out seem remote from this country. Nevertheless some of the readers of the articles might be misled into thinking that that they represent mainstream Christianity. It is strange that unbelievers want Christians to believe the most alarming doctrines, and often seem themselves to disbelieve in a God that has never been worshipped by any Christian of my acquaintance! However we feel about it, our patients are not coming to us with a fear of hell, nor is a hospice a place to exercise, far less to preach, judgement. Lingering fears there may be, but that is all they are for the great majority of folk.

Jesus, quoting Isaiah, spoke of the bruised reed, which was not to be broken, and the flickering taper, which should not be extinguished.[5] I would like to propound a 'bruised reed' theology of palliative care. Such sparks of spiritual life as there are, such memories of childhood teaching as persist, should be encouraged and affirmed in our patients. It is just too easy to want to correct, to teach and to argue, and hospice patients are usually too tired and weak to think bright new thoughts. Yet there is goodwill towards the church, and seldom hostility. There is a basis of faith, often like a grain of mustard seed, on which to build. Perhaps that is all changing, as the generation that was sent to Sunday School and the men who grew up in the Boys' Brigade diminishes.

John was a young man from an outlying part of Edinburgh, an area which is sometimes described as an area of urban deprivation. He had no recent connection with the Church. Nor did his wife. Yet, after a few weeks, he confided in me that he and his wife read the Bible and prayed every night. Perhaps he had been brought up in the church, and something or someone had disillusioned him. He did not say. And I wonder how many people keep up the practice of private religion without 'benefit of clergy', Grace Davie has famously written of 'Believing without Belonging'.[6] John certainly wanted a Christian funeral. He represents a fair number of folk who believe but not in the institutional Church. Such people are not very satisfactory supporters of the hard-pressed local clergy and their buildings and projects, but they have chosen their privatized version of Christianity, and it must be admitted that for some it works.

So palliative theology will be non-judgemental, and will rejoice in fragments of faith. Kathleen was judgemental. She knew the truth, but she was sure that no one else did.

She went to church, but constantly criticized her minister, theologically and morally. No one was like her grandfather, a clergyman whose example she kept always before her. She had built a spiritual wall around herself. What could the chaplain do, as she faced her death – not at all with equanimity? Story-telling, remembering, common acquaintances were shared, and gradually from behind the façade emerged a real and sad person, who confessed feelings of inadequacy and failure, and who began to have a glimpse of the mercy of God.

The mercy of God, his unconditional love, his self-giving in Christ, are all themes in this palliative divinity. Cicely Saunders, in many of her writings, has suggested that we cannot know how the Holy Spirit will work in the hearts and minds of dying people. I have had to learn that I am not the last line of defence. God has other servants, who might be listening while on night duty, or when they are cleaning under the bed, or cutting hair. And when he does not use human agency he is not bound by his normal means of revelation. So I can be optimistic about patients and their relationship with their maker. Otherwise I could not sleep.

You may think that I am making heavy weather of this. Do chaplains not simply deliver what patients want, without regard to their own faith? Of course we must operate in a professional way, and not favour one believing patient over another who is not interested. But surely it is not possible to be possessed of a living faith, and be indifferent to the predicament of others. It is needful to have a wide view of the working of God, and a firm faith in his love to continue this work with integrity.

These insights, like the discoveries about medication made by trainee doctors, must be reflected in the wider areas of the minister's work. As the worshipping church continues to decline in numbers, perhaps chaplains have a mission to remind the faithful and the unfaithful of the unbounded wonder of God's love.

LITURGY IN A HOSPICE

St Columba's Hospice has had a succession of chapels, and

chapels are there to be used. The chapel is open for anyone to visit and sit quietly, thinking and looking out of the window, or talking intimately in a measure of privacy. Its main function is for worship. It is only too easy to import practices from outside. I have dealt in detail with some experience of worship in the hospice in a previous chapter. Here it is important to stress that this is a place of learning and experiment. There have not been secular and multi-denominational hospices before the last part of the twentieth century, and now they can be a testing ground for worship. Should only well known hymns be sung? Or can the resources of contemporary Christian song-writing be used? Is it possible to deal with New Testament passages which promise healing to faith, or tell of miracles of recovery and the raising of the dead, or ought the reader to choose more bland readings? Should there be a set order for morning prayers, or can each leader choose her own style? These questions have been faced, but never ultimately decided.

It may be of interest to sketch the order of communion which was worked out over a number of years, and used each Sunday afternoon, strictly between 4.30 p.m. and 5.00 p.m., so that the patients were not late for tea:

1 Welcome and explanation, sometimes necessary because most Sundays there were those patients, families, and volunteers present for the first time.
2 Hymn. Both the *Church of Scotland Hymnary* and a Catholic hymnal were in use.
3 Prayer and Lord's Prayer.
4 Scripture, followed by a very brief homily.
5 Communion. The usual rite was an adaptation of the Order for Home and Hospital in the current *Book of Common Order* of the Church of Scotland. The bread was taken to worshippers in their seats or sometimes in their beds, and followed by wine from the common cup. Prayers of intercession were included in the communion prayer.
6 Hymn – if there were enough present!
7 Prayer and Blessing.

Occasionally exception was taken to the common cup, but by

volunteers, never by patients. In the Church of Scotland and other Protestant churches it is more usual for the wine to be served in small individual cups. A tray of these was hidden in the vestry, but never used.

This brief service of word and sacrament was no doubt capable of modification and improvement, but was for most participants familiar enough so that the strangeness of the setting did not obtrude. There were those who stayed away because the service was advertised as communion, but in my experience, more were attracted than repelled. An invitation to communion always contained a recognition that some present would prefer not to participate.

After the service communion might be taken to patients who were not well enough to attend, and who requested a visit. Sometimes a prayer at the bedside seemed appropriate. Sometimes it seemed right just to tell the story. Sacraments are central to hospice worship, and what has been almost a routine becomes much more full of meaning and much more productive of emotion in such a setting. Communion became, I believe, a 'converting ordinance' in some cases.

Because it is possible to see some matters more clearly in a small institution, I believe that there are lessons to be learnt by the churches from the hospice experience. In particular the doctrinal and ecclesiastical barriers which we argue about with such vigour when we are with the healthy seem to matter less in face of death. If death is an ultimate test of faith and also a place of revelation, then hospice discoveries must not be dismissed as the experience of a chosen few.

FOR FURTHER THOUGHT

1 What right has a chaplain to impose her own religious ideas on others?
2 Is it possible to research the meaning and effects of religious belief?

NOTES

1 Russell Stannard, *The God Experiment*. London: Faber & Faber 1999, pp. 1–12.
2 Organized by one Derek Doyle!

3 Tony Walter, *The Eclipse of Eternity: a Sociology of the Afterlife*. Basingstoke: Macmillan 1996, p. 25.
4 Boyd C. Purcell in *American Journal of Hospice and Palliative Care* (May/June and July/August 1998).
5 Matthew 12.20.
6 Grace Davie, *Religion in Britain Since 1945: Believing Without Belonging*. Oxford: Blackwell 1994.

CHAPTER SEVEN

The Hospice as Problem

Only a few years after the great Dedication service at St James, Anytown, disaster struck. The Governors, great and good citizens of Anytown, resigned *en masse*. There had not been a financial failure, or gross misbehaviour. They had simply realized that the hospice had moved beyond their perceptions, had invited researchers and students, had become 'just another hospital' as one of them put it in a letter to the local newspaper. He was able to quote a nurse who had been there from the beginning who said that she had not come to a hospice to nurse geriatrics.

The general public perception of the hospice movement is that it is a great blessing to humanity and that to be cared for in a hospice is a good thing. Attempts to change its name because of another perception of a hospice as a place only for dying have foundered on the fund-raising possibilities of a familiar title. 'Specialist Palliative Care Unit' does not have quite the same ring about it when the cans are rattling in the High Street. Hospices have quite rightly traded on their place in public goodwill, and as more and more families benefit from them, so the goodwill spreads. In Edinburgh consistent funding by the public has survived a special appeal from the Sick Children's Hospital, and the setting up both of an AIDS Hospice in the city and a Children's Hospice not far away. Generosity seems almost limitless, and if funds are carefully managed the mixed economy of state and charitable funding has been seen to be effective.

The danger with new ventures is that they become established and then they are not open to being changed. There occurs a 'routinization of charisma'. What begins as a prophetic sign is welcomed into an unreformed or unreformable existing system. What begins as a counter-cultural enterprise becomes part of the culture that it has set out to criticize. As doctors in the community and in the hospitals come to rely on the hospice to manage certain of their patients, they begin to expect to lay down the terms for admission. As the National Health Service helps to finance the hospice, its managers want, rightly, to know what the policy is and how the money is being spent. As the unit becomes more and more part of a larger community system, its religious roots can become obscured and the Christian ethos less prominent. It is difficult to distinguish between what is inevitable and what can be modified.

Let me give an illustration from outside the hospice world. Many years ago a Children's Holiday Village in the country near Edinburgh was converted into a home for children with learning difficulties. It was very successful in its first two decades, and was run on strong evangelical Christian principles, by a leader who had a remarkable rapport with the residents and their families. But as they grew up the residents continued to be treated as children, and were given very little responsibility for themselves. Their lives were restricted to a very safe environment, and most of the parents and the voluntary supporters of the venture were happy with this. Then the leader died, and those who succeeded her lacked her charisma. Money was taken from the Social Work Department, but its norms were not followed, and eventually inspectors stepped in, and an appalling situation discovered. Another Christian agency took over, not without great difficulties, and the now middle-aged residents live in small family units, travel independently, have their own rooms and are even allowed to watch television, something that was previously banned. It is a venture that in its early years achieved great things, but it lost its prophetic edge, and was fortunate in its rescue.

Hospices are always in a very delicate situation. They must not conform entirely to old ideas about the care of the dying, and they must not lose their calling to provide good care. But there must be research and teaching; buildings need to be updated; there are demands for standards set by outsiders who may not know, or may not seem to know, much about hospices.[1] This 'routinization of charisma' (Weber's phrase) of which researchers write[2] seems to be inevitable as the generation of pioneers passes on. Those who were willing to go against received public opinion and raise both awareness of the needs of the dying and money for the implementation of their vision eventually have had to retire, and their places have been taken by financially astute committees and highly qualified palliative care professionals. Recent research into the work Dame Cicely Saunders carried out in the 50s and 60s suggests that she was aware that this would happen, and was able to face the possibility with equanimity.[3]

Nevertheless the evolutionary changes in the hospice concept are bound to have effects on spiritual care. Cicely Saunders insisted on spiritual care as an integral part of all 'holistic' care. When this demand becomes institutionalized it is in danger of becoming a subtle form of patient control. Just as the 'stages of dying' theory associated with Kübler-Ross has been sometimes uncritically adopted as a template for all patients, so spiritual responses come to be measured and applied in a way that deprives the patient of her individuality. The glorious muddle of dogmatic, religious, and folk beliefs that make up the spirituality of many people is put into a defined series of statements and entered on a spiritual needs chart, and the patient is categorized on a religious/spiritual scale. Now this is possibly an exaggeration, but there is a real danger of losing spontaneity and sensitivity as routinization progresses. As palliative care becomes part of the wider medical knowledge, so its special status is threatened.

Along with routinization and secularization came the concept of medicalization. There has been much illuminating thinking on the developing status of medicine in society, as recent scientific advances seem to have taken authority from religion and the churches and transferred it to the medical establishment. Ivan Illich maintained that much illness was in fact iatrogenic (i.e. resulting from a generalized societal dependency on medical intervention). Birth and death moved from the home to the hospital until it began to be considered wrong to give birth or to die outside a medical context. Hospices were sometimes thought of as providing an alternative to this modern trend, and to be returning to a more holistic and 'wise' way of dealing with advanced illness. With the gradual development of palliative medicine has come, some would argue, an intensive medicalization of the whole movement.[4] This has turned it into merely an adjunct of the National Health Service. Illich certainly states his case well, and on a worldwide canvas, and some of his ideas have influenced popular thinking. Definitions of sickness and the assumptions of power by the medical world have been questioned, and it has been noted recently that the general esteem for doctors has declined, not least because of horrific cases of medical malpractice. Yet the medical model of caring for the dying prevails in hospices, and seems to have been only marginally challenged by the existence of multidisciplinary care teams. All students are treated equally, but preference in the allocation of space and time is given to medical students, allegedly because their courses are much more crowded.

Organizational structures continue to grow, management becomes more hierarchical, and rules displace immediate responses. Much of this is of course necessary and inevitable. The 'amateur' status of early days was also sometimes inefficient. The selection of staff and volunteers was occasionally influenced more by the willingness of those offering their services than by the perception of their proven skills. A group of enthusiasts working together, supported by a committee of well-wishers in the community, was not an edifice that could survive the investigation of Health Boards and the scrutiny of the public press. When money was sought from the National Health Service, then the application of standards became inevitable. Criteria were set and protocols introduced. Increasing emphasis on training has produced highly qualified nurses, without the feared loss of commitment to people. Nurses still come to hospices to carry out 'real nursing' as they have envisaged it, so that they can have time to talk to patients, and to share some of their own personality with them.

In the field of hospice chaplaincy there has also appeared an element of professionalization. Whereas typically clergy saw themselves as being 'called' to their work, received a stipend and not a salary, and saw their chain of command going through church structures to God himself, we are now being caught up in more human chains of command, and we have stopped being ashamed of having professional skills. Structures of responsibility have been set up, with many chaplains managed by Directors of Nursing, and a few by medical directors or social workers. New duties, such as the co-ordination of paramedical services, have been added to the purely ministerial and pastoral functions traditionally expected. Skills in counselling and management are demanded of some new appointees, and courses have evolved where the necessary training and learning is offered and carried out. The University of Glasgow offers a multidisciplinary Diploma and an MSc. degree in Palliative Care, and several clergy have taken advantage of this. The University of Leeds offers a BA degree in Chaplaincy, and at Lampeter, Reading and other universities there are courses on various aspects of death and dying.

Clark and Seymour caution against too easy acceptance of the theories of routinization and medicalization, and point out that 'the conscious decision to make religion secondary to medicine within the St Christopher's project led to the spreading hospice movement being a community of religious motivation which could engage with the secular world of healthcare and service organisation.'[5]

FUNDING

The problem of the intermediate status of the hospice gives rise to other questions. If state funding is to be accepted, how much control must be given away? If the hospice still relies largely on voluntary contributions, how are these to be managed? Hospices are open on the one hand to the criticism that they use scarce resources for an elite group of patients, and on the other that they rely too heavily on dubious methods of fund-raising. It is not my intention to become involved with the complex arguments concerning the National Lottery. I do know that many hospices have applied for grants, and that some have been successful, especially for the funding of new units and other capital projects. Others, mindful of their religious origins, and of the sensibilities of many religious people, have not yet applied. With the ready acceptance of the Lottery, and the evident use of at least some of its profits for excellent causes, any principled opposition to it as a form of gambling which Christians should avoid may seem to be mean-spirited. But I do see a real dilemma here which I fear will be resolved on purely utilitarian grounds. Recently the hospice which I know best has started a Prize Draw scheme, and it remains to be seen how its more puritanical and Protestant supporters will perceive this.

Lesser games of chance, raffles and such, are already accepted as legitimate forms of fun and fund-raising, but even here there are residual signs of opposition. My father, a confectioner by trade, was persuaded to give a demonstration of cake decorating to the Day Hospice patients and staff. The leader suggested that the cake should be raffled and I had to point out that my father with his strict evangelical views would be absolutely horrified! I think the cake was cut up and eaten. But he is not alone, and questions about ethical fund-raising will continue to arise in broader or narrower contexts.

THE LIMITS OF ACCEPTABILITY

What happens to people with other long-term illnesses? At one early stage hospices were seen as suitable places for sufferers from multiple sclerosis, cerebral palsy and other long-term conditions, but it was soon realized that care for acute cancer patients put a particular burden on nurses and doctors that could not easily be combined with the different needs of those with chronic conditions. The Leonard Cheshire Foundation and other agencies are particularly adapted to the care of those who might be expected to live for a number of years.

In the mid 1980s, when Edinburgh earned the unenviable title of 'the AIDS capital of Europe', one of the areas most affected by the results of needle-sharing was quite near St Columba's and there was much discussion of the possibility of being more open to accepting HIV-AIDS patients. As it happened, Milestone AIDS Hospice was opened at the other end of the city, and it was possible to point to it as the appropriate place for care. But other factors were involved. The HIV-AIDS affected and infected population was on the whole younger, had distinctive life-styles, and had a very uncertain prognosis, which made it difficult to contemplate care being given in one institution both to cancer and to AIDS patients. Certainly among the patients admitted with terminal cancer there were some who were HIV infected, but the policy decision not deliberately to accept HIV-AIDS patients was taken. In subsequent years the whole picture has changed, with the use of new drug regimes, and the recent partial withdrawal of funding from the AIDS Hospice. This is an unfinished story, and experiences have been different in other hospices.

THE VEXED QUESTION OF EUTHANASIA

In Jalland's fascinating book *Death and the Victorian Family*[6] we meet Dr William Munk, a devout Roman Catholic whose book named *Euthanasia; or Medical Treatment in Aid of an Easy Death* (published in 1887) provides a guide to the care of the dying endorsed by the highest medical authorities of the period. He uses the word 'euthanasia' in the classical sense of 'a calm and easy death'. Much space is given to advice on the alleviation of pain and distress, and he is anxious to dispel the popular belief that pain was both inevitable and beneficial to the dying person, whose mortal struggle and death agony were so vividly and frequently portrayed in fiction and in evangelical literature as enviable. Munk recommended the use of opium as a pain relief, and the wise provision of alcohol. The patient should be allowed to express wishes about diet and stimulants. In many ways Munk anticipated the work of twentieth-century specialists and his work remained authoritative for over thirty years. Thereafter it seems to have been forgotten and some of his principles began to be rediscovered in the 1960s.

In 1902 Dr Robert Saundby of Edinburgh discussed euthanasia in *Medical Ethics: A Guide to Professional Conduct*. He
defined it in clearly modern terms as 'the doctrine that it is
permissible for a medical practitioner to give a patient suffering from a mortal disease a poisonous dose of opium or other
narcotic drug in order to terminate his sufferings'. This would
be contrary to the fundamental rule that doctors must hold
human life sacred, and take no action which would deliberately destroy it.[7]

So much for the development of the concept. It is sad that
the basically kind word 'euthanasia' should now be applied to
non-natural death. But we must accept the language as it is.
There has been a continuous debate for many years about the
possibility of legalizing voluntary euthanasia, and many references have been made to the Netherlands, where very
recently, in 2000, the law has caught up with medical practice,
and euthanasia, within very strict conditions, has been
decriminalized. In the Northern Territory of Australia a brief
experiment of legalizing euthanasia was brought to an end by
federal legislation, and in Oregon, USA, a form of euthanasia
has been allowed.

In the UK the Voluntary Euthanasia Society has led the
demand for the legalizing of some form of mercy-killing, gaining much popular support, and being concerned in several
so-far unsuccessful attempts to change legislation in Parliament. It is clear that this is a subject that will not go away,
and since good hospice care has been adduced as a powerful
anti-euthanasia argument, it will be necessary to review the
matter. There are many areas of the discussion where boundaries are unclear, and an attempt at definitions is necessary. I
follow the chapter by Oxenham and Boyd in *New Themes in
Palliative Care*.[8] They usefully set out definitions:

- The term *euthanasia* should be reserved for the 'compas-
  sion-motivated, deliberate, rapid and painless termination
  of the life of someone afflicted with an incurable and pro-
  gressive disease'.
- Euthanasia is *voluntary* if it is performed at the dying
  patient's request or with that person's consent. If it is

performed without a person's consent it is *non-voluntary*;
If against a person's consent it is *involuntary*.
- *Treatment-limiting decision* is a description of any action
  concerning withdrawing or withholding treatment which
  is deemed to serve no purpose, even if life is shortened.
  This is generally held to be ethically correct. This description has replaced the terms *active* and *passive euthanasia*,
  which are ambiguous and should be avoided.

Occasionally in the course of a terminal illness a drug used to
control a symptom is thought to contribute to or hasten the
death of a patient. This treatment can be justified by the
principle of *double effect*. Relieving, by appropriate measures,
a patient's pain and suffering even if it shortens life is not
euthanasia.[9]

Felicity was a highly intelligent woman who until she contracted cancer had led a charmed and happy life. Her sense of
humour never deserted her, and so I cannot be sure how serious
she was when she asked to be 'put down', as she phrased her
desire for induced death. 'Nurses and doctors could all stand
round me in my bed and one could give the injection. No one
would know who had done the deed.' Next morning her
jokes were less macabre. Many patients have asked to be
killed when in the grip of despair, only to remark the next
day, 'Cancel that conversation!' More often it is relatives who
suggest that their loved one should be put out of agony.
Sometimes much persuasion is needed to ensure that they
believe that pain is under control, and that the patient is
indeed in some sense comfortable.

Every hospice must have anecdotes on this theme, and one
constantly asked question is 'Do you practise euthanasia?'
The answer is always negative, not least for legal reasons. But
the questions and demands require a more nuanced response.
It is too simple to say that as Christians or as hospice workers
we are against euthanasia. What is being done when a patient
is heavily sedated, and becomes effectively dead to his family,
with only minimal response? Some families go home and do
not return until called in. Others watch lovingly or with dread
for the slightest signs of response, and stay until the end. We

could keep some people alive longer, by treating all infections, by subcutaneous fluids, or by other means. But there is a time to die, and it not the hospice's business to keep alive by extra-ordinary means, unless there is a good reason, such as the imminent arrival of a daughter from New Zealand.

It might be assumed that Christians are entirely against euthanasia, but just as there are a number of positions on the lawfulness or otherwise of abortion, so there are about the end of life. Until recently the Chair of the Voluntary Euthanasia Society in Edinburgh was a retired Bishop of the Episcopal Church of Scotland. In *A Dignified Dying*[10] Hans Küng and Walter Jens discuss the parameters of mercy-killing, and put great stress on dignity in dying.

In several publications[11] the Anglican theologian Paul Badham has argued positively for a Christian acceptance of a form of euthanasia. He remarks that for many Christians the question of euthanasia is a non-issue, decided in advance by Pope or evangelical teaching. It is simply wrong. 'It does not help that strong support is given for euthanasia by the British Humanist Association who have claimed that it is extremely hurtful to require someone who does not believe in God or afterlife to suffer intolerable pain or indignity in deference to a God or afterlife he does not accept.'[12]

Badham points out that Christians have changed their attitudes to medical discoveries, and takes as an example the gradual acceptance of anaesthesia after Queen Victoria had accepted the use of chloroform in childbirth. The churches which had been vehemently against the reduction of natural pain gradually changed their minds. Many Christians have been strongly opposed to contraception, but the majority of Anglicans and Protestants would no longer take that stand. Badham argues tentatively that medical advances, while removing many pain-based reasons for euthanasia, have also provided new possibilities of autonomy in the face of death. He points out that the Bible is at the least ambivalent about suicide, that Jesus exalts laying down one's life for others, and that there is a long tradition in the church, from the days of the early martyrs, of willing acceptance of death, which need not represent the last enemy to Christians. In some cases euthanasia could be seen as a self-chosen acceptance of God's will, and arranging the time of one's death would give the opportunity for a dignified, and indeed a holy leaving of this life. The ideal death of fiction and piety might indeed be achieved if, after receiving communion and saying goodbye to family and friends, a person could then die at peace with his fellows and with God. This brief summary scarcely does justice to Badham's argument, but it might serve to show that not all Christians always decry euthanasia.

Of course there are powerful counter-arguments, concerning the sanctity of life, the principle of human autonomy, and the very practical consideration that dying people change their minds when they are feeling better, or after a good sleep. Advance directives to family or doctor, drawn up when a person is well and alert, do not necessarily reflect the mental position and the will of that same person suffering a terminal illness. My own belief is that the great majority of people cling fiercely to life, however it is hedged about with physical and emotional limitations.

For a chaplain the question is quite often posed in a modified form by patients, usually but not always elderly, who are, at least on the conscious level, impatient to die. Jessie was one such. She was an active member of her church, and made sure that everyone knew this. But one day another woman with the same name died in the ward. Jessie's hard-to-answer question was 'Has God made a mistake? Or have I offended him in some way?' For a long time she was inconsolable. What can one say to this question? If an older person has made his peace with God, is reasonably content that life is completed, is weary and unable to keep up any interests, is it any wonder that he begins to doubt God's providence? Facile remarks about heaven being not quite ready scarcely help, but sometimes asking if there is a significant event or anniversary coming soon may suggest an explanation of the delay of death.

In our changing society it is certain that the question of euthanasia will not go away. Hospices are involved in the debate, and must ensure that their response is carefully argued and incapable of being dismissed as dogmatic and unthinking. There will be changing expectations about death, especially in an atmosphere that emphasizes choice, and in an increasingly secular milieu. Reports on the situation in the Netherlands vary depending on the viewpoint of the reporter, and there is certainly an interest in developing hospice care there. Some have seen it as a counter-influence to the practice of euthanasia in that country, but it is surely better to emphasize the ability of palliative medicine to remove in many cases the need for artificial termination of life.

Practice in hospices needs to be constantly reviewed lest we seem to do what we condemn. Does the administration of sedative or analgesic drugs hasten death or not? Can we be sure either way, and can we always take refuge in the principle of double effect? We aim to care for the patient in every way, and there is a very fine line between allowing to die and hastening death by medical means. There is a constant need for information and for the education of the public in what hospice care can and cannot do, indeed must not do, whether that is prolonging life with no good reason or deliberately shortening it. Essential is the maintenance of trust, and openness in communication. This is a subject that will continue to recur.

SPIRITUAL HEALING

To pass from the vexed question of euthanasia to what sounds like a fad or fringe movement may seem a little abrupt. But faith healing, healing by spiritual persons or means, healing that does not conform to medical science, so far as it is certain, is not a remote subject in hospice work. Kay had found the news of life-threatening cancer very hard to accept. She was quite young, active and felt that there should be a great deal of life in front of her. Nominally Catholic, she sent for the priest, who gave her the sacrament of the sick. She was anointed and prayed for[13] and nothing much changed. She continued weak and exhausted, and her mind was certainly not at rest. She heard of a Pentecostal church where healings were said to take place. She attended for a few weeks, finding the worship atmosphere somewhat strange, and the pastor prayed, laid on hands, and proclaimed her healed. But she was not, nor was she very reassured. Soon she came to the hospice as an in-patient. An outspoken woman, she roundly condemned both attempts at healing, and submitted to the hospice routine, eventually dying with some measure of peace. Kenneth, on the other hand, always claimed to have been helped by the many healing agencies and services which he travelled far and wide to attend. Sometimes the healing was done by post, and sometimes the ceremonies were in Kenneth's home. Perhaps he went to a church, but I do not think so. Travel and love-gifts became expensive, and his family resources were limited, yet he continued to claim that it was all worthwhile. He died a disillusioned man. Margaret was a sharp young businesswoman who was found to have breast cancer when she was nursing her first child. She belonged to a strong Christian family, and had put her financial acumen to work for the church she loved, a church which might have been described as middle-of-the-road and fairly liberal. When she was ill, she made no secret of her condition, and various well-meaning friends drew her into a healing group, where she began to pick up the message that it was her lack of faith that hindered a complete cure. Perhaps this was an inverted form of hope, perhaps she was exhibiting symptoms of deep guilt. Certainly her situation was full of problems. She refused to see her own pastor, and made her parents most uncomfortable. I wish I could report that the matter was resolved before she died, but I cannot. The healing group acted according to their beliefs, and might not have blamed Margaret as she thought they did. There is a desperation in some patients, especially those who are younger, which sends them to any source that offers healing, and if it is within the church, so much the better, or possibly the more dangerous.

Here is one more example. Clare had been a missionary for many years. She and her husband were now retired, which meant that they continued to run prayer groups and address meetings all over the country. When she was admitted to the hospice she was anorexic and weak, and she was liable to pathological fractures of the bones. Her husband and a group from their church, including the pastor, an old friend of mine, gathered around the bed and prayed that she would be healed. I was told that there were groups in many parts of the world sharing the prayer and hope, and that the longer the cure took to perform, the more people would be convinced of the power of God. The nursing staff were very unhappy at the situation and were sure that the family's faith would crumble under the weight of unreal expectations. But when Clare did die, her husband praised the Lord that she had been taken to glory. His theology was not so rigid, nor his expectations so focused as we had feared. There was a lot of talk about this among the staff for some time, when the chaplain felt that his role was as interpreter of evangelical religion to Christians of other traditions. As Clare had served as a missionary in France, the situation was especially puzzling to Catholic nurses!

Some healing prayer groups have proved to be of great help to patients. They have supported the patient and family, have not intruded on treatment, and have taught the uncertainties of treatment and outcome, while maintaining hope. There are many who can testify to the power of prayer in time of illness, and there seems to be no doubt that illness goes far beyond the physical realm and that there are areas which are mysterious and impossible to define. It is those groups which put guilt on the patient, or assume it themselves, which can lead to problems. Healing crusades, of which there are many in all parts of the world, can keep seekers away from recon-ciliation with the will of God by falsely raising hopes of what may be possible. The progress of advanced cancer may be stopped for a time, but in the end it is inexorable. Neither prayers nor exorcisms can remove the tumour or stop the spread of metastases. But trust can bring spiritual calm and acceptance.

The churches have always believed that it is right to pray for health and healing, and there is a variety of liturgies and practices available. Prayer for the sick is part of the normal life of the church, and anointing and the laying on of hands in a context of faith and acceptance is to be encouraged. Promises of instant cure, if enough faith is exercised, or the right words said, are of quite a different order. Occasionally patients are advised to refuse medication, and healers, secular as well as religious, can undermine the work of doctors. It is a matter of some delicacy to determine whether such counter-cultural healers should be allowed to visit, yet if there is a long-standing relationship between healer and patient, that relationship should not lightly be terminated. We touch here on an area of mystery, and an area where faith and scientific medicine can clash, and a hospice is a place where this conflict can be observed and sometimes resolved.

ALTERNATIVE OR COMPLEMENTARY THERAPIES

There have always been conflicting schools of medical thought and practice, and allopathic medicine happens to be that endorsed by authority and the majority of people in Britain. Alternatives have been seen as at best unorthodox and faddish, and at worst dangerous. Homeopathy, aromatherapy and reflexology have gained a certain amount of respectability in recent times, and there is a Chair of Complementary Medicine in at least one English university.

In hospices there has been some resistance to complementary therapies, possibly because in the public mind hospices themselves have been seen as alternative ways of providing care, and hospice doctors have been anxious to be considered as mainstream orthodox practitioners. It is partly the mystique of the hospice which has given rise to the misapprehension that it is in some measure part of the 'New Age' group of healing arts. I have felt both the suspicion of those who are wary of 'New Age' and the interest of those who are involved in it in some way. So there is a narrow path to be followed. Certain therapies, such as hand massage with aromatherapy oils, have been found to be helpful. Acupuncture for the control of pain, and hypnotherapy for the relief of stress and fear have both been practised at different times in hospices. The National Council for Hospices and Specialist Palliative Care Units has an ongoing group studying the subject. Patients accustomed to alternative therapies should certainly not be denied access to them when they enter a hospice, but it is an open question whether the unit has the right to introduce patients to different ways of care. Diets, whether self-chosen or imposed by religious beliefs, must be honoured, however inconvenient for the kitchen staff. Hospices are surely small enough places for personal preferences to be honoured.

OTHER FAITH COMMUNITIES

It is impossible, even in quiet country places, not to be aware that the United Kingdom is even more than in the past a mixture of communities. Celts, Angles, Saxons and Norsemen at least share a Christian heritage. The Jews have been settled since Cromwell's time, and even most of those who came from central Europe in the nineteenth and twentieth centuries consider themselves reasonably acculturated. The difficulties they have faced in becoming involved with hospices have been ideological. Sometimes the movement has seemed to take away hope and that is contrary to Jewish faith. Yet discussions and explanations have broken down barriers, and the North London Hospice, in particular, has catered for many Jewish patients and has had two rabbis from different schools as chaplains.

There are other problems for Muslims, Sikhs and Hindus, who do not seem to make as much use of hospices as their numbers warrant. The hospice movement has theoretically no credal or racial bounds. But it is still perceived by many from our ethnic communities as white, middle-class and Christian. Home care services are more called upon, and it may still be true that smaller communities are better at looking after the sick at home. Yet this will change as new generations, born here, adopt more Western norms of social behaviour. The hospice movement needs to listen to our minority people, and indeed to those seeking asylum, and it may be that this will change the ethos of many institutions. As more receive higher education, strategic posts will be open to those who do not share all the ideals of the founders. Perhaps the chapel will have to be renamed, or other prayer rooms provided. In the mean time, respect for traditions and customs which may seem strange to Westerners must be taught and practised. Most Muslim and Sikh families will make their own arrangements with their religious leaders, and it is necessary to appreciate that ideas of pastoral care might be quite different from Christian or secular practice.

SEX AND DEATH

How many hospices have rooms with double beds? Not all our patients are old, nor does disease kill all desire. The need to be held closely by a loved one may increase in the last days of life. We are always told that it is important for carers to touch patients, to hold hands and stroke brows and never to pull away in obvious distaste from even the most disfiguring tumour. That is true, and every pastoral worker must be taught to act on her own instinct to be tactile. There is appropriate touching, and there is inappropriate. I think that we have been too quick to rule out intimacy between couples as undesirable and too difficult to arrange, or as slightly shocking 'in his condition'. Privacy to celebrate an anniversary with a special meal, or for a family birthday party, is not too hard to organize, and it has been touching to be told that 'that was the best anniversary we've ever had'. Hospice kitchens are good at producing birthday cakes. But may a wife or partner spend the night in the patient's bed? Why not? The patient has often been cared for at home until admission, and the warmth of loving contact should not be automatically withdrawn. Certainly it is difficult. How can interruptions be avoided? What will other families say? But it is certainly worth considering. There could be a room with a larger bed.

Sex and death make a potent mixture, as P. D. James, among many others, remarks.[14] In *Death, Desire and Loss in Western Culture*[15] Jonathan Dollimore traces the intimate connection in different phases of our culture between the desire to live and the necessity of death. From Shakespeare to Freud the theme is pursued. A hospice is on one level a clinical environment where good care of sick people takes place. On another it is full of strong emotion. There can be an almost frantic need to cling to life when the extinction which death brings threatens us. This can affect staff working with the dying, who can be heard to say, 'I must live every day as if it was the last.' It can puzzle partners who are not involved in the same work. There is a certain desperation that sometimes affects us, and it is as well to recognize it.

THE DARK SIDE OF HOSPICE CARE

Too often hospices are portrayed, especially in their own literature, as places of light and hope, where noble deeds are done and great victories won. Certainly there are many instances of good care and renewed faith, and many patients have received help beyond what they have expected. It would be dangerous, however, to rely entirely on the words of grateful users. Those who work in hospices are not angels, nor are they more devoted and skilful than those who work in the National Health Service or in nursing homes. Ambition, rivalry, mixed motives, even lapses in concentration are there, as they are anywhere else. Spending so much time with dying folk and their relatives must affect staff at quite deep levels. There can be a culture of black humour which seems to be a necessary antidote to the surrounding gloom. Patients can be seen as objects of experiments as well as real human beings. The higher the ideals and claims put forward, the harder it is to live up to them. Yet in my experience there have not been many examples of burn-out, partly because staff have often been able to see when it is time to move on, and partly because of good peer-support in a relatively small institution. Great care is also taken in selection. Constant exposure to grief in all its forms can make us callous, yet life and experience call us back to our humanity. It has to be stated that the pressures of hospice work do produce casualties, yet the movement does not seem to have been in existence long enough for research to be done on long-term effects. What there is points to the prevalence of human weakness, and the remarkable results nevertheless obtained.

In her book *The Dying Process*, to which I have already referred, based on research in a hospice which was undergoing morale-destroying problems, Julia Lawton writes of the experience of patients who have lost control of the body's physical boundaries, who have suffered in her words 'the sequestration of the unbounded body'.[16] She instances a patient whose bodily deterioration caused offensive odours, of which the woman seemed to be oblivious. As the patient wished to remain in a shared room, the smell caused problems for other patients, and for the staff, whose best efforts to control the situation were unsuccessful. Eventually she was transferred to a single room, where her condition was such that her family stopped visiting, as they considered her beyond their reach. It is a sad story, not so much of the failure of hospice care, as of the fate of humans with eroding tumours, and it could easily be multiplied.

Hospice care does not remove the unpleasant effects of cancer. Odours can be controlled but not eliminated. Families and other visitors can leave feeling sick and angry and defeated, and staff can feel that their work is impossible. Patients can be overwhelmed by shame when they become incontinent – or they can be cheerfully oblivious to their loss of control. It does the image of hospices no favours to hide these facts.

Just as difficult are the instances of what Lawton calls 'social death'.[17] Sometimes patients do not deteriorate as quickly as they would like, or as their relatives expect. Susan came to the hospice with a very short prognosis, but in the warmth and care of the room she stabilized, and indeed began to take notice of her surroundings. Her family had assumed that hospice meant imminent death and had emptied her house and handed the keys back to the council. They were quite appalled to learn that she might soon be able to go home, because now there was no home, and when Susan found this out she was inconsolable. She was alternately angry that she was still alive, and furious with her family for considering her dead. She remained with the hospice, full of grievance until mercifully her condition altered and in a few days she died, still unreconciled either to her death or to her family. Sometimes there is no right answer to, and certainly no explanation for, the dying process.

There are other disconcerting forms of behaviour which are hard to contain in the 'perfect hospice' ideal. Patients may have had episodes of mental illness in the past, and react in unexpected ways to care and treatment. The illness may affect the mind or the brain and a patient may embarrass her relatives with her language, or her attitude to the nurses. Sheer frustration and boredom may drive a person to extreme actions. Occasionally a patient tries to escape from the building, and sometimes family collude. When Philip could bear the hospice no longer, he went out through the front gate in his pyjamas and dressing gown, accompanied by his sister, who seemed to think that this was a normal thing to do. He was brought back and once safely in bed, he admitted to his anguish. Indeed boredom is one of the great enemies to be overcome. Patients attempt the crossword every morning, and when it becomes impossible for them, as their mental acuity diminishes, they can be difficult to console. Some patients bring books, and can be seen to read the same page for several days. In fact reading and any form of entertainment that requires concentration is difficult, because treatment and visitors and cleaners and mealtimes interrupt the fragile sense of normality. It must be hard to sit and stare if one has been active with hands and mind, and sometimes the best efforts of diversional therapists can make little difference.

'What is going through your mind as you look out at the garden?'

'Nothing. I just want out of here.'

A cure for boredom would be a good palliative weapon. Jolly conversation, jigsaw puzzles, or simple knitting may not always be the answer. When pain is at last controlled, and nausea is dispelled, what is the tired weak patient to do but sleep? And that might mean lying awake at night, when everything seems so much worse.

Perhaps hospices raise as many problems as they answer.

FOR FURTHER THOUGHT

1 Should hospices look to a future when they have done their task?
2 Is there a cure for boredom?

NOTES

1 The story of the new Health Service managers who pointed out to hospice management that they seemed to have an unusually high death rate and asked how they were going to remedy this is surely apocryphal!

2 David Clark and Jane Seymour, *Reflections on Palliative Care.* Buckingham: Open University Press 1999, pp. 107ff.
3 *Op. cit.*, p. 119.
4 Ivan Illich, *Limits to Medicine: Medical Nemesis, the Expropriation of Health.* Harmondsworth: Penguin 1977, pp. 179–211.
5 Clark and Seymour, *op. cit.*, p. 119.
6 Pat Jalland, *Death in the Victorian Family.* Oxford: Oxford University Press 1996, pp. 83ff.
7 *Op. cit.*, pp. 93–4.
8 David Clark, Jo Hockley and Sam Ahmedzai, eds., *New Themes in Palliative Care.* Buckingham: Open University Press 1997, pp. 275–87.
9 *Op. cit.*, p. 276.
10 Hans Küng and Walter Jens, *A Dignified Dying.* London: SCM Press 1995. Cf. also Hans Küng, *Eternal Life?* London: Collins 1984, pp. 187–218.
11 Paul Badham in Paul Badham and Paul Ballard, eds., *Facing Death: an Interdisciplinary Approach* (Cardiff: University of Wales Press 1996), pp. 101–16; also Paul Badham in Robin Gill, ed., *Euthanasia and the Churches* (London: Cassell 1998), pp. 41–59 and subsequent discussion chapters.
12 Quoted from the Select Committee on Medical Ethics, in Paul Badham, *Facing Death,* p. 102.
13 James 5.
14 P. D. James, *Original Sin,* London: Faber & Faber 1994, p. 82: 'The potent conjunction of death and sex, I suppose.'
15 Jonathan Dollimore, *Death, Desire and Loss in Western Culture,* London: Allen Lane The Penguin Press 1998.
16 Julia Lawton, *The Dying Process: Patients' Experiences of Palliative Care.* London: Routledge 2000, p. 124.
17 *Op. cit.*, pp. 150ff.

CHAPTER EIGHT

Moving On

It is scarcely possible to escape from the subject of funerals and their conduct. There is a story that whenever clergy get together they tell stories of graveside disasters and crematorium adventures. Be that as it may, to work in a place where sooner or later people die is to be made to think about the function and meaning of funeral rites.

Almost all cultures have developed ceremonies, rites and stratagems for disposing of dead bodies. There is evidence from neolithic times of special treatment of the dead, and the monuments of a succession of civilizations have left the countryside with many signs of funerary practice. From the Great Pyramids of the Pharaohs on the edge of Cairo, to the barrows and chamber tombs of England, from the Necropolis that overshadows Glasgow Cathedral to the most remote country burial ground, mementoes of death and of what happens to the remains of dead people are always with us.

The assumption that the Christian dead should be decently interred in the earth, and in hallowed ground, was challenged at the end of the nineteenth century, when the overcrowding of urban graveyards was becoming a problem, hygiene was much considered, and dogmatic Christian views about death and burial were waning. Gradually the idea that cremation was an acceptable, clean and decent way of disposing of remains was accepted by the majority of people in Britain and increasingly in Continental Europe and North America. In 1986/7 70.5 per cent of funerals in England and Wales were cremations, 55.6 per cent in Scotland, 42 per cent in Holland and only 15.2 per cent in the USA.[1] Each religion has its own regulations, and Jews and Muslims are still usually interred, and Hindus are cremated. Very conservative Protestant Christians resist the idea of cremation for various reasons. Some argue that the body must be in one place in order to be reconstituted at the Resurrection; others that cremation was practised in biblical times by pagans, and that the early Christians, like their Master, were buried in the earth. Another interesting argument in favour of burial is that a gravestone leaves a testimony to faith, if it is suitably inscribed, while the tiny memorial tablet at the crematorium, or the rosebush in the garden of rest, is not designed to speak of the glory of God and the shortness and uncertainty of human life. Certainly historical researchers and genealogists would find their work much more difficult without funerary inscriptions.

For most people, Christian and post-Christian, in our urban society, cremation has come to be the normal way of disposal. In country places, where graveyards are not yet filled, burial remains the majority choice. Occasionally families argue about what Father really wanted, but most folk make their wishes clear. The invention of the crematorium and its chapel, so relatively recent in our long human history, has given rise to much thought among clergy and others who have to lead the services there. Wherever they are conducted, funerals are final and they are not repeatable. So it becomes one of the duties of a chaplain to conduct them well, if she is called upon to do so. Opinions vary on the part a hospice chaplain should play in this. There are those who argue that as a person has lived in a community, so the departure from life should be marked in that community, and conducted by the local incumbent, even if that person has not known the deceased. If it is neighbours and friends who will attend the funeral, then someone familiar to them should be there so that there can be community mourning and the local people can give support to the bereaved. Hospice chaplains have no direct role here, and should contact local clergy in almost all cases, unless the dying person has especially asked for their services. In an ideal situation there is a lot to be said for this attempt to assert the interest and the continuing life of the parish.

Despite this desire for the ideal, what so often happens is that the person who dies in the hospice has had no real connection with the local church of whatever denomination, and the relatives and carers are quite widely scattered in the immediate community and far beyond. If there has been a church connection, however tenuous, then the local minister may well be the right person to be contacted, and certainly if there is church membership, then there is no question about who normally would be expected to conduct the funeral. But, if, as so often happens, the only 'holy' person who has had any contact with the deceased is the chaplain, then she is the obvious person to be asked to conduct the service. Certainly the relatives may be confused, or feeling guilty for neglecting the deceased, and less than fully aware of what the choice is, when they visit the funeral director, and certainly some funeral directors are more directive than they ought to be. Yet it is important for families that the service is conducted by someone who 'knows' the patient, rather than by a 'rent-a-rev' hired by the funeral director, or by the hitherto unknown and probably overworked parish minister.

The tentative approach of a patient's daughter, when she realizes that her mother will soon die, is very important, and must be honoured. The circumlocutions are many, but eventually the request comes. 'If anything happens to my mother, will you say the good words?' Occasionally a patient asks outright. 'Do you do funerals?' To which the response has to be: 'Yes, of course – have you told your family?' It is important to many families to know that the conductor of the funeral is not just inventing the tribute, but has taken notice of what the relatives have said, and has at least actually seen the person who has died. This may seem obvious, but it needs to be underlined. I believe that hospice chaplains have a right to conduct funerals if they are asked so to do, and that they also have a duty to the family to make a local pastoral connection if that is possible. Sadly, it seldom is, not least because so many families are scattered, but from time to time it has worked, and a real connection with the church has been forged.

As has been said, the funeral service, wherever and by whomever conducted, is a once only event, and must be carefully planned and sensitively performed. Perhaps not many of the words spoken are exactly remembered, even by the nearest kin, but the attitude, the tone of voice, and the approachability and manner of the officiant make an impression. A rushed service, or one conducted without apparent interest, will be remembered as a bad experience, as will one when the name of the deceased is not mentioned.

Fergus spent about three weeks in our hospice, gradually becoming at the same time more comfortable and weaker. He had definite views about his funeral, which he made clear to his family and to the chaplain. 'I have been a very important person, and I want it to be done properly, for the sake of my reputation among those who attend.' And indeed he must have been quite notable, judging by the great and the good who appeared at the crematorium on Christmas Eve. He had his social position to uphold, and he indicated he was not opposed to Christianity, which at least made a start in preparation for the service. The funeral was a social event, a fitting ending to a successful career.

When James's wife died he came to me in distress. 'Joan was an atheist and she wanted no minister at her funeral – but what will the neighbours think?' I felt it my duty to point him to authorized humanist officiants. Funeral rites differ in various parts of our country and among denominations, so that it is difficult to generalize about them. The experience of the hospice points to the continuing importance of the service, both to mark the passing of an individual, and to consolidate and possibly relieve the grief of the family. It is a rite of passage, and cases where a funeral cannot be held, for example when no body has been recovered, leave relatives in a continuing state of uncertainty. It is of course the right of any person to give instructions that no public funeral service be held.

In the United Kingdom a smaller percentage of babies are baptized than in the past, fewer people are married in church, but most funerals are still conducted by a minister. It is our chance to be important to the family for a very brief but crucial time. Gathering information about the deceased, whom the chaplain may have met only in his last illness, is important and requires tact and the ability to see through conventional language. It is still not acceptable to speak ill of the dead, yet the temptation to idealize needs to be resisted. The most that family will usually admit is that their old father was stubborn, or that he liked the betting shop and the pub. References to these interests can raise a knowing smile at the service, and such pursuits are part of the authentic person whom it is now obligatory to celebrate. Only occasionally has a widow allowed herself to show relief, or retrospective anger, when her husband has died, but I am convinced that many more in different relationships to the deceased would have liked to express some sort of pleasure at the death.

There still seems to be a belief that only ministers can and should conduct a funeral, whereas there are no legal requirements as to who should carry out the service. Family or friends may conduct the service and give the eulogy. The spread of the custom of asking a friend to speak at the service, even when a minister conducts it, has been attributed to the influence of popular culture, in particular to scenes in soap operas. On the one hand this is to be welcomed, as it takes away from the minister the necessity of speaking eloquently about someone she has scarcely known, but on the other there is the danger of inordinately long tributes, and the possible embarrassment when emotion overcomes the speaker.

Should then the minister conducting the funeral be honest to the point of pointing out the flaws in the character of the deceased? It seems to be expected that the prayers will be comforting, the hymns old and familiar, and the tribute fulsome. Yet the best compliments are, 'You just got him right,' or 'You sounded as if you knew her.' These are scarcely fulsome and I have had at the back of my mind for some years a comment from a priest in a letter to the press: 'When we are told that that was a good funeral what is really meant is that it was not as bad as it might have been.'[2] In the past a funeral was a time to proclaim the gospel, and the liturgies of all churches contain strong references to the resurrection. But more and more the emphasis is on a eulogy on the deceased. This is in line with the modern emphasis on the value of the individual, and the place of the biography of the deceased in bereavement theory. The focus has shifted, even in the funerals of believers, from the proclamation of the mysteries of the faith to the celebration of an individual life, within the relationships of the family, the workplace and the church.

There have also been changes in the music and poetry thought appropriate for funerals. Chaplains will have their own convictions about their authority to sanction or refuse modern songs, such as 'My Way' and readings such as 'Death is nothing at all'.

Funerals are and ought to be an important part of the work of the hospice chaplain. They require time and sensitivity. She will be dealing with people at their most vulnerable, and also their most receptive moments. She might find herself in strange and sometimes scary family gatherings, or conducting long-distance telephone conversations to prepare a meaningful and personalized version of eternal verities. Sometimes she will be asked to perform the rite as part of the hospice package. Since the nurses are kind and the doctors competent, it is assumed that the chaplain will know what she is about. This compliment to hospices can be accepted gratefully. When the Medical Director asked me in what part of my work I felt most confident and competent I answered 'funerals' without thinking much. The minister is briefly important, she is doing what no other friend can do, and she is in charge!

Funeral rites are changing. In some ways there is a return to what is perceived as traditional. In Edinburgh, at least one large firm of funeral directors maintains a horse-drawn equipage which is increasingly being asked for. Directors now walk in front of the hearse for a short distance, top hat in hand, from the house where the deceased lived, and again at the approach to the crematorium. This is surely a deliberate attempt to slow down the proceedings, and to offer a mark of respect. On the other hand I have noticed very few men, in recent years, removing their hats as they watch a funeral procession from the roadside. Perhaps that is because it is no longer fashionable for men to wear hats, but it can also be attributed to a lack of respect for the dead. More often impatient car drivers cut through the line of mourners' vehicles. Funerals are deeply important for those involved, but decreasingly marked by such public gestures as drawing curtains in neighbouring houses. This change has been praised as it reminds us not of gloom but of hope in the time of death. Nevertheless I believe that it is a sign of a wish not to dwell on such a morbid matter. It is the chaplain's task to help mourners to balance hope with sadness, and to try to strike the right balance between the ministerial role of proclamation and pastoral sensitivity to the feelings of those she is serving at a particularly tense time.

BEREAVEMENT

Bereavement is another much discussed topic in recent publications. Consolation for the grieving has always been the responsibility of ministers, and it has also been the task of close relatives and friends. To visit the bereaved is a difficult but necessary task, and its omission by a minister is long remembered. Letter-writing is said to be becoming a lost art, but letters of condolence are still written and much appreciated by the bereaved person. When my wife died I was quite overwhelmed by the number and content of the letters I received and I resolved to be more diligent in writing to grieving friends. Even when we are more familiar with telephone and e-mail we turn to letters to express our grief and solidarity. It is less immediate, and we can take our time about it.

There is a long and honourable tradition of letters of consolation. Jerome[3] writes to console his friend Heliodorus on the death of his nephew Nepotian. He contrasts human despair or resignation with Christian hope, he gives a eulogy of the departed both as man and presbyter, and he then reviews the evils besetting the empire, from which an early death has removed the young man. Christian consolation has become a lament for a dying world. Calvin[4] in a letter to Viret whose wife had died strikes a refreshingly pastoral note.

Come to Geneva on this condition, that you disengage your mind not only from grief, but also from every annoyance. Do not fear that I will impose any burden on you, for through my means you will be allowed to take whatever rest is agreeable to you. If anyone proves troublesome to you, I will interpose.

Ariès writes of consolation literature in America:

> the letter of condolence is a classical genre that was culti-
> vated as much in antiquity as in the Renaissance and the
> seventeenth century and was related to the elegy, the liter-
> ary tombstone and the epitaph. In nineteenth century
> America the genre, once intimate, became public and the
> nature of the arguments, the tone and the style changed
> completely. The titles are suggestive: *Agnes and the Key of
> her Little Coffin* (1837), *Our Children in Heaven* (1870). The
> authors of these books were clearly obsessed with the
> images and ideas of death.[5]

Ideas of the afterlife portrayed in such consolatory literature have moved from the theocentric and christocentric views of the New Testament, the Fathers and the Reformers to a much more anthropocentric description.

Pat Jalland in *Death in the Victorian Family* looks at a wide range of letters of consolation and charts the gradual shift from scriptural admonitions to a much more secular tone.[6] Most such letters today are private. There are how-to-do-it books giving formal instruction, and recently *A Book of Condolences*,[7] giving a wide variety of examples from many religious and literary sources, has been published in the United Kingdom.

According to Tony Walter death as loss has in the twentieth century come to supersede the idea of death as passage, and the psychologists have taken over from the theologians. He recalls that Anglican students whom he interviewed were more at home with the psychology of bereavement than with the doctrine of the resurrection. CRUSE, he claims, is suspi-cious of counsellors with too firm a belief in the orthodox doctrine of the life after death, which may get in the way of sympathetic listening to the bereaved person's own experience of loss.[8]

Certainly I did not find the letters which were mainly con-cerned to state Christian hope as comforting as those which contained personal stories and came from friends of very varying forms of belief and unbelief. For better or worse bereavement care now concerns not dogmatic avowals of faith in the resurrection but a real engagement with an individual's story. CRUSE conforms to this in that it is, or was in its origins more than thirty years ago, a self-help organization devoted to meeting the needs of widows and widowers. It has developed a well trained group of counsellors, but remains in essence an organization which is chosen, not imposed.

Many hospices have bereavement services, taking various forms. Typically they are in the hands of social workers and chaplains, with perhaps input from a clinical psychologist. That may involve monthly meetings in the hospice or on neutral ground of those bereaved folk who wish to take part. Home visits are often undertaken. Those who attend are encouraged to share their experiences and difficulties and are also offered personal support. There is no doubt that such activities help many folk. It is important not to feel alone, or that this has never happened to anyone else. It is good to find a listening ear. There are problems. Some become unhealthily dependent on the group and have to be gently discouraged from further attendance. Some are too inarticulate to wish to be in a group. Some come back to the hospice and are disappointed that their favourite nurse is not on duty. Some may use a group to make new relationships. But insofar as hospices seek to care for the family as well as the dying person, a bereavement service of some kind seems to be a necessity.

Services of thanksgiving and remembrance are held in many places. It seems necessary for some to come back to the hospice one last time, to say goodbye and to make an effort to begin again. Again, there has been a varied response to such gatherings. Catholics are accustomed to requiem masses, and to celebrating the anniversaries of a death. Protestants are less used to this. Yet a great variety of the bereaved do attend a quarterly service, sometimes coming in family groups, and often meeting up with other families in the same situation. St Christopher's Hospice has tried to find out how many nonbelievers attend, and what the reaction of various groups has been. There have been attempts to offer a secular meditation, and in other places a service complete with hymns and a sermon has been the chosen mode. No such service will please everybody or cater for all needs, but many appreciate the opportunity to remember someone they have loved in a familiar place. More local churches are also holding annual remembrance services, either at All Saints at the beginning of November, or at Easter.

Such events and organizations can temper grief, but they cannot completely take away the pain and the longing that assail the bereaved. Nor can they deal with the unexpected memories that are stirred by quite trivial sights and sounds and even scents. The classical grief theory which has prevailed in Western society basically argues that the 'proper' relationship between the living and the deceased is a severing of ties and a form of reintegration, which usually involves entering into new relationships. So the emphasis has been on 'moving on', 'letting go', resolving grief by detachment from the past. This is so brief an account as to be something of a caricature, but there is plenty of literature which gives a more coherent and nuanced account.[9]

In the first number of *Mortality* Tony Walter propounded 'a new model of grief: bereavement and biography'.[10] He has expanded on this in his recent book *On Bereavement*. He urges that the bereaved should be encouraged to talk about the deceased, to construct a biography, and to incorporate them into ongoing life. He suggests that this has implications for funerals, and for bereavement counselling. Officiants have a duty to learn as much as they can of the lifestory of the deceased and to use that knowledge in their service, and counsellors should give bereaved people permission to seek out and talk to those who knew the deceased. In this way, far from becoming detached from one another, the living can retain real links with the dead. This approach attracts me, and in the context of the hospice stresses integration rather than detachment, surely a hospice motif.

Various strategies have been suggested to maintain bonds. Pictures and writings have long been in use. Modern technology might allow recordings of messages, and videos, to go alongside dreams, imaginary conversations and prayer. What has been dismissed as dangerous, namely a preoccupation with the dead person, can now be seen as useful and healthy. Pathological grief will still occur, and will need expert help, but the lines between good and bad grief are less well marked and there is room for more research.

FOR FURTHER THOUGHT

1 How helpful can a counsellor be if he has not known the deceased?
2 How can funerals be improved? Does hospice experience contribute any insights?

NOTES

1 Tony Walter, *Funerals and How to Improve Them*. London: Hodder & Stoughton 1990, p. 22.
2 Source now unknown.
3 Nicene and Post Nicene Fathers, second series, vol. 6, p. 123.
4 *Letters of John Calvin*. Edinburgh: Banner of Truth Trust 1980, p. 83.
5 Philippe Ariès, *The Hour of Our Death*. London: Allen Lane 1981, p. 450.
6 Pat Jalland, *Death in the Victorian Family*. Oxford: Oxford University Press 1996.
7 Rachel Harding and Mary Dyson, eds., *A Book of Condolences: from the private letters of illustrious people*. London: Azure 1999.
8 Tony Walter. *The Eclipse of Eternity: a Sociology of the Afterlife*. Basingstoke: Macmillan 1996, p. 122.
9 See, for example, Colin Murray Parkes, *Bereavement: Studies of Grief in Adult Life* (Penguin 1980), and the writings of J. William Worden.
10 Tony Walter in *Mortality* 1:1 (March 1996), pp. 7–26.

CHAPTER NINE

The Hospice, a Sign of Hope?

There are many ways to characterize the last few decades. Observers have commented on the individualization and the privatization of life in the West. The solidarity which was evident in British life after the Second World War, and which in part gave rise to the welfare state, has given place to a prosperity which has produced consumerism, selfishness, a growing gap between rich and poor, and a decline in civic virtues. People seem less willing to join any sort of organization, and not only churches but also the great political parties show a steep decline in membership. The results of what can generally be called post-modernism have made us suspicious of the grand narrative, and that includes the health narrative of the NHS.

In contrast to this stands the hospice movement. This has been a faith-based initiative, with old-fashioned values which owe much to concepts of Christendom. It has a firm volunteer basis, and finds little difficulty in co-ordinating voluntary and professional services. It stands for compassion and operates within a small-scale framework. While there are bodies such as Help the Hospices and the National Council for Hospices and Specialist Palliative Care Services which seek to co-ordinate work in the area of palliative care, and an Association of Hospice Chaplains which has begun to look for international links, and while there are many journals and textbooks, each hospice has continued to claim a certain independence. Government requirements to set and monitor standards have eroded the possibility of hospices behaving just as they like and have also made it necessary to define what the hospice is.

Nevertheless local committees and some financial indepen-dence as well as a common commitment to ideals of care have given identity to otherwise diverse institutions. Hospices have shown that it is possible to be effective without being large, and they have also made it clear that a higher ratio of staff to patient can be maintained, with accompanying bene-fits. They have also become places of research and discovery, so that the care, particularly of patients with cancer, has been noticeably improved. In co-operation with other cancer char-ities, especially with the Macmillan Cancer Relief Fund, some progress has been made in reducing the effects of cancer.

The future of hospices has been much discussed. Their evolution from Christian homes for the dying to today's more secular institutions is inevitable. To that extent hospices are not immune from the spirit of the age. In recent years fewer free-standing units have been built, and there has been a great extension of community palliative services to cover most of the United Kingdom. Small hospice wards have been built into the structures of some larger hospitals, and palliative care teams set up within other hospitals. One can only speculate what this will mean for more traditional hospices. Already a few have had to close completely or in part, and others have financial strains to struggle with. Possibly smaller hospices will amalgamate and share such services as chaplaincy. The bigger and the more efficient and adaptable units will endure, and grow in public esteem. The time for a hospice heritage trail has not quite arrived.

THE HOSPICE AND THE CHURCH

If the hospice movement has a prophetic function in society at large, and possibly in the world of medicine, does it still have a message for the Church which so largely gave it birth? It is trite to say that the institutional Church is in decline. Believing without belonging is more common than devoted church membership, and Callum Brown has alarmingly charted the 'Death of Christian Britain'.[1] Undoubtedly the church-centred culture of the earlier twentieth century which Brown describes in great detail is much attenuated, and the Christian faith no longer so overtly shapes public opinion and behaviour. What Brown says as an historian is underlined by the churches' own surveys, such as *The Tide is Running Out*, compiled by Peter Brierley.[2]

Prophets and prophetic institutions are not easily integrated into establishments. The Old Testament prophets were opposed and persecuted, and sometimes paid for their stance for truth with their lives. They were also strange, angular, uncomfortable characters, whom we would not invite home for dinner. Jesus the prophet of Nazareth told the rulers and the rich home truths which thoroughly discomforted them. We cannot expect to be considered a prophetic movement without conflict, going against received opinion, and raising quite vocal opposition. Nor can we pursue our calling without making mistakes, hurting and being hurt.

Many people are interested in God and spirituality, but have been damaged by the institutional Church. They have been ignored, devalued and condemned, or so they believe. Church buildings have closed, congregations have migrated, and they themselves may live far from the familiar streets where they grew up. Yet longings are there and they are stirred to life when death approaches. It is good that some are reconciled to the church when they are in a hospice. Perhaps this is the equivalent of the Victorian deathbed conversion. But it is sad that so many seem to be missed by the church on the corner.

From the standpoint of a hospice chaplain I have seen much that is good in the practice of the church. Many clergy are assiduous and skilful in visiting the dying. Some are clearly uncomfortable and might do more good by sending a sympathetic layperson. Some congregations have excellent pastoral networks, and teams of visitors for the sick and bereaved. Others work in a more haphazard way, and leave too much to the stipendiary minister. Hospices are one of the agencies where experience and training are available for clergy and congregations in the care of the dying, and they ought to be open to welcoming groups and individuals who want to learn more.

Even the most open church practises some form of exclusivity. No single congregation can suit all tastes and convictions. A hospice is open to all in need, and has to learn tolerance and

co-operation, not only among Christians, but also across religious divides, and between believers and unbelievers. With
their Christian roots, perhaps hospices are in a unique position to show one way forward to the churches. They can have
a prophetic voice, not looking back to a golden age when
everyone went to church, for there never has been such a
time, but looking out to the many people who have spiritual
longings which Christians believe are only met in Christ.

A SPIRITUALITY OF HOSPICE CARE

In her book *The Spiritual Care of Dying and Bereaved People*,
Penelope Wilcock writes:

> Terminal illness mounts a serious attack on the sense of
> identity. The powerlessness, loneliness and fear commonly
> experienced feel dehumanising and alienating, and consti-
> tute (or trigger) spiritual crisis in many people. It is hard
> to believe in a God who cares, who is merciful and offers
> security, in a life situation where all that was reliable and
> familiar is disintegrating, where one's home territory is lost
> and the new environment is not home.[3]

To reassure, to comfort and at the same time to be truthful is
the task of the spiritual carer. Too many have false or unex-
amined ideas about God, and in a hospice setting many
patients are weary and frightened. If the loving and forgiving
God in whom Christians believe can be made evident – for he
is present – by those who wash and clean and converse with
and listen to the dying, then great good may be done. Alastair
Campbell writes:

> Ministry is offered whenever one person becomes the ser-
> vant of another in his search for faith. This service may
> consist of sacramental acts, of preaching, of private conver-
> sation, or of simply being present to the other in a shared
> silence. In all these activities the minister is a servant in the
> sense that he offers whatever he has to the other to meet
> the other's need. (This is not to deny of course that he also

receives much in return.) Thus ministering to the dying is in essence sensitivity to what each individual is going through in this particular crisis. There are no special techniques to be learned, no routine questions to cover one's own anxiety, no one attitude that will fit every situation.[4]

I believe that hospices are in an early stage of development, and that there is much more to discover about human reaction to death and dying. Spiritual care, however defined, must continue to be central to planning and staffing. Roland Riem, in his moving book *Stronger Than Death*, writes:

> If patients cannot always abandon themselves to their dying in the fashion of the saints, the same can also be said of pastors in their ministry... Pastors too fail in their witness to the truth, sometimes through lack of courage or detachment, sometimes because their strength or faith fails them. Yet they will still be able to witness to the light.[5]

I hope that in this book, which I realize has had many personal touches in it, I have been able to convey a sense of the light and shade of hospice ministry, and to witness to the love of Christ.

NOTES

1 Callum G. Brown, *The Death of Christian Britain: Understanding Secularisation, 1800-2000*. London: Routledge 2000.
2 Peter Brierley, *The Tide is Running Out: What the English Church Attendance Survey Reveals*. London: Christian Research 2000.
3 Penelope Wilcock: *The Spiritual Care of Dying and Bereaved People*. London: SPCK 1996, p. 66.
4 A. V. Campbell in Derek Doyle, ed., *Terminal Care*. Edinburgh: Churchill Livingstone 1979, pp. 58-9.
5 Roland Riem, *Stronger Than Death: a Study of Love for the Dying*. London: Darton, Longman & Todd 1993, p. 106.

Further Reading

A short and necessarily arbitrary list of books, out of many that could have been listed, for further reference and study.

Ainsworth-Smith, I. and Speck, P. *Letting Go.* New edition, London: SPCK 1999.

Ariès, P. *The Hour of Our Death.* Harmondsworth: Penguin 1983.

Badham, P. and Ballard, P. (eds), *Facing Death: an Interdisciplinary Approach.* Cardiff: University of Wales Press 1996.

Bailey, E. I., *Implicit Religion in Contemporary Society.* Kampen, Netherlands: Kok Pharos 1997.

Becker, E., *The Denial of Death.* New York: Free Press 1997.

Bowker, J., *The Meanings of Death.* Cambridge: Cambridge University Press 1991.

Campbell, A. V., *Rediscovering Pastoral Care.* London: Darton, Longman & Todd 1981.

Cassidy, S., *Sharing the Darkness.* London: Darton, Longman & Todd 1988.

Cobb, M. and Robshaw, V. (eds), *The Spiritual Challenge of Health Care.* Edinburgh: Churchill Livingstone 1998.

Hick, J., *Death and Eternal Life.* London: Collins 1976.

Hockey, J., *Experiences of Death.* Edinburgh: Edinburgh University Press 1990.

Lawton, J., *The Dying Process: Patients' Experiences of Palliative Care.* London: Routledge 2000.

Lyall, D., *Counselling in the Pastoral and Spiritual Context.* Buckingham: Open University Press 1995.

Riem, Roland, *Stronger Than Death: a Study of Love for the Dying.* London: Darton, Longman & Todd 1993.

Rumbold, B. D., *Helplessness and Hope: Pastoral Care in Terminal Illness.* London: SCM Press 1986.

Walter, T., *The Eclipse of Eternity: a Sociology of the Afterlife.* Basingstoke: Macmillan 1996.

Walter, T., *The Revival of Death.* London: Routledge 1994.

Walter, T., *On Bereavement.* Buckingham: Open University Press 1999.

Wilcock, P., *The Spiritual Care of Dying and Bereaved People.* London: SPCK 1996.

Index